Liver Cirrhosis and Its Complications - Advances in Diagnosis and Management

Edited by Ran Wang and Xingshun Qi

Published in London, United Kingdom

Liver Cirrhosis and Its Complications - Advances in Diagnosis and Management
http://dx.doi.org/10.5772/intechopen.111135
Edited by Ran Wang and Xingshun Qi

Contributors
Ali Husnain, Ali Sepehrinezhad, Ali Shahbazi, Cai'e Wang, Chuanfang Chen, Hongyu Li, Jing Chen, John Fung, Lei Chen, Ning Kang, Osman Ahmed, Ran Wang, Shubei He, Ting Wang, Wali Badar, Xiaozhong Guo, Xingshun Qi, Ying Peng, Zhenyu Wu

First published in London, United Kingdom, 2024 by IntechOpen
IntechOpen is the global imprint of INTECHOPEN LIMITED, registered in England and Wales, registration number: 11086078, 167-169 Great Portland Street, London, W1W 5PF, United Kingdom

British Library Cataloguing-in-Publication Data
A catalogue record for this book is available from the British Library

Additional hard and PDF copies can be obtained from orders@intechopen.com

Liver Cirrhosis and Its Complications - Advances in Diagnosis and Management
Edited by Ran Wang and Xingshun Qi
p. cm.
Print ISBN 978-0-85466-392-7
Online ISBN 978-0-85466-391-0
eBook (PDF) ISBN 978-0-85466-393-4

For EU product safety concerns:
IN TECH d.o.o., Prolaz Marije Krucifikse Kozulić 3, 51000 Rijeka, Croatia,
info@intechopen.com or visit our website at intechopen.com.

Meet the editors

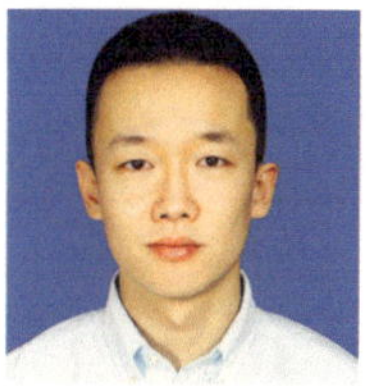

Dr. Ran Wang is the attending physician of the Department of Gastroenterology, General Hospital of Northern Theater Command, China. His major research interests include the etiology, diagnosis, and management of liver cirrhosis, portal hypertension, and portal vein thrombosis. He is a committee member of the Liaoning Immunology Society, Liver and Immunology Subdivision.

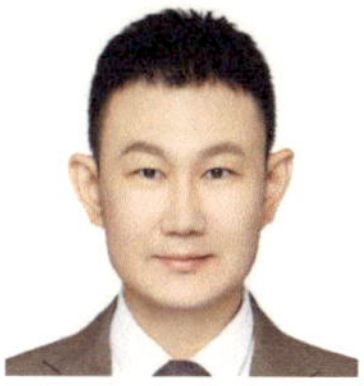

Prof. Xingshun Qi is the director of the Department of Gastroenterology at the General Hospital of Northern Theater Command, China. His major research interests are the management of liver cirrhosis, portal hypertension (especially portal vein thrombosis and Budd–Chiari syndrome), and hepatocellular carcinoma. He has edited nine English-language books and serves as a senior editorial board member for *BMC Gastroenterology*, an associate editor for *Frontiers in Medicine*, an academic editor for the *Canadian Journal of Gastroenterology and Hepatology*, an editorial board member of *Therapeutic Advances in Gastroenterology*, and an editorial board member of *Advances in Therapy*.

Contents

Preface

Liver cirrhosis represents the end-stage of multiple chronic liver diseases, characterized by a deteriorating prognosis and a heavy health burden *Liver Cirrhosis and Its Complications – Advances in Diagnosis and Management* provides a comprehensive review of the latest advancements in the diagnosis and management of liver cirrhosis and its associated complications.

This book is structured into six chapters, each offering in-depth insights into critical areas of liver cirrhosis. These chapters encompass discussions on the diagnostic methods and therapeutic strategies for cirrhosis, the utilization of transarterial radioembolization (TARE) therapy for hepatocellular carcinoma, the pathology of hepatic encephalopathy, and the clinical applications of non-selective beta blockers (NSBBs) in cirrhosis management.

The book integrates a wide range of perspectives, from clinical to pathological, and features contributions from esteemed authors worldwide. This multidisciplinary approach ensures a robust understanding of the progress made in diagnosing and managing cirrhosis and its complications. This book provides readers with novel perspectives and innovative approaches, ultimately contributing to the enhancement of diagnostic and therapeutic practices for liver cirrhosis. By addressing current gaps in knowledge and practice, this book aims to significantly advance the field of hepatology and improve patient outcomes.

On a personal note, I would like to express my deep appreciation for the support of my family, whose encouragement has been invaluable throughout my work. Special thanks to my wife, Ms. Mengzhu Li. Despite the challenges you have faced, your perseverance continues to inspire me, and I believe brighter days are ahead. I extend my heartfelt gratitude to my mentor, Professor Xingshun Qi, for his unwavering support and guidance in both my professional and personal life. His mentorship has profoundly shaped my career, providing opportunities that have made me who I am today. I am deeply grateful for our encounter and look forward to contributing even more to our field in the future.

Ran Wang and Xingshun Qi
Department of Gastroenterology,
General Hospital of Northern Theater Command,
Shenyang, China

Chapter 1

Introductory Chapter: Liver Cirrhosis – Innovations in Diagnosis and Management

Ran Wang, Xiaozhong Guo and Xingshun Qi

1. Introduction

Liver cirrhosis is the end-stage of various chronic liver diseases, frequently caused by viral hepatitis, chronic alcohol abuse, non-alcoholic fatty liver disease, autoimmune liver disease, genetic diseases, and cholestatic liver diseases. Liver cirrhosis is a significant health burden globally; it is currently the 9th cause of death in Europe and South East Asia, representing the 15th leading cause of disability-adjusted life-years globally [1]. Early diagnosis and management of cirrhosis and its complications are imperative to improving outcomes for individuals with cirrhosis. Our research group has consistently focused on the diagnosis and treatment of liver cirrhosis and its complications, achieving significant progress in various aspects. These efforts and work provide a solid foundation for inviting experts worldwide to collaboratively write this book and share the newly developed innovations in the diagnosis and management of liver cirrhosis with the readers.

2. Non-invasive diagnostic methods in esophageal varices

Gastroesophageal varices (GEVs) appear in approximately 50% of cirrhotic patients and represent one of the most prevalent and severe complications of liver cirrhosis [2]. Acute variceal bleeding is a major cause of death in cirrhotic patients. Despite the advancement of treatment strategies, variceal bleeding is still associated with a 6-week mortality rate of 15–20% [3, 4]. Upper gastrointestinal endoscopy is the gold standard for diagnosing GEVs. However, it is an invasive procedure, complicated with poor patient's tolerance. Recent studies have demonstrated significant progress in the non-invasive diagnosis of GEVs.

Our research indicates that traditional non-invasive markers for assessing liver fibrosis have limitations in predicting esophageal varices (EVs) [5]. In contrast, scoring systems based on clinical laboratory results may be more helpful for the non-invasive diagnosis of EVs. Therefore, we innovatively developed the Liaoning scoring system. Qi et al. created the Liaoning score from a group of prospective cirrhotic patients who had their first endoscopy at 11 hospitals in Liaoning Province, China [6]. A total of 363 patients with cirrhosis participated in this study, of whom 71.63% (260 out of 363) had EVs. EVs were independently associated with acute upper gastrointestinal bleeding (AUGIB), platelet count, and ascites. In cirrhotic patients, the Liaoning score had an area under curves (AUC) of 0.807 ($p < 0.0001$). With a cutoff value of 0.474, sensitivity was 70%, and specificity was 77.67%. This study found that Liaoning score, a new scoring system, can predict EVs in cirrhotic patients. Li et al. externally validated the Liaoning score in a nationwide multicenter cross-sectional study for EVs and high-risk EVs prediction [7]. A total of 612 cirrhotic patients with AUGIB participated in this study. The incidence of EVs and high-risk EVs was 96.2% and 95.6%, respectively. The results revealed that the Liaoning score's AUC for predicting EVs was 0.708 ($p = 0.0016$), and that of high-risk EVs was 0.702 ($p = 0.0147$).

Computed tomography (CT) plays an important tool in assessing complications of cirrhosis and screening for hepatocellular carcinoma. Our study findings support CT's potential in non-invasive diagnosis of EVs. Contrast-enhanced CT was utilized in a study by Li et al. to predict GEVs non-invasively [8]. A total of 279 patients were enrolled in this retrospective study. High-risk varices, which include EVs and gastric varices, are defined as varices requiring treatment. Based on endoscopic surveillance, drug prophylaxis (primary or secondary prophylaxis), and history of bleeding events, all patients were categorized into four groups. Only contrast-enhanced CT was significantly correlated with EVs, high-risk EVs, and gastric varices in the general population. The cutoff value of high-risk EVs was determined to be a diameter of less than 0.5 cm, less than 0.38 cm, less than 0.46 cm, and less than 0.33 cm for the primary prophylaxis, acute bleeding, previous bleeding, and secondary prophylaxis populations, respectively, which avoids 47.8%, 10.5%, 12.1%, and 7.8% of endoscopic surveillance without high-risk EVs. This study demonstrated the high diagnostic accuracy of contrast-enhanced CT in patients with GEVs.

3. Management of portal vein thrombosis in liver cirrhosis

Portal vein thrombosis (PVT) is a common yet complicated complication that affects approximately 10–25% of cirrhotic patients [9]. Most cases are asymptomatic and diagnosed during routine screening. Some studies have even suggested the transient nature of PVT [10]. However, acute symptomatic PVT can precipitate a rapid deterioration in cirrhosis. Anticoagulation therapy stands as a primary treatment for PVT. Recent research confirms the efficacy and safety of anticoagulants in managing PVT in cirrhotic patients [11]. Analysis from 33 studies and 1696 patients highlights that anticoagulation therapy significantly boosts portal vein recanalization rates ($RR = 2.61$) and survival ($RR = 1.11$), without notably increasing bleeding risks ($RR = 0.78$). Early initiation of anticoagulation is particularly effective, enhancing recanalization ($RR = 1.58$). Direct oral anticoagulants (DOACs) are shown to be safer in reducing major bleeding events ($OR = 0.55$) compared to traditional anticoagulants, across 29 studies involving 2469 patients [12]. Gao et al. examined the role of thrombolytic therapy in PVT treatment through 29 cohort studies and 131 case reports or series [13]. The results indicate that early initiation of thrombolysis is effective, with a 58% rate of complete recanalization. However, the benefits may be reduced in cases of PVT secondary to acute pancreatitis, highlighting the importance of careful patient selection. These consolidated data support personalized, evidence-based management of PVT in cirrhotic patients, recommending anticoagulation and DOACs based on individual risk profiles. Early thrombolytic therapy may prove effective, but requires further validation through additional high-quality studies.

4. Prognosis assessment in cirrhosis

The assessment of prognosis in patients with liver cirrhosis is of critical importance for clinical management, as it facilitates the identification of high-risk individuals who may benefit from early liver transplantation and aids in the formulation of personalized treatment plans. Additionally, prognosis assessment facilitates the formulation of personalized treatment plans by clinicians and the ongoing monitoring of disease progression.

Peng et al. evaluated Child-Pugh, MELD, and ALBI scores for predicting in-hospital mortality in cirrhotic patients with acute-on-chronic liver failure [14]. The AUROCs were 0.63 for Child-Pugh, 0.75 for MELD, and 0.53 for ALBI, indicating marginal effectiveness in predicting outcomes. A similar study on acute upper gastrointestinal bleeding (UGIB) in cirrhosis [15], involving 145 patients, showed AUROCs of 0.796 for Child-Pugh and 0.810 for MELD scores, suggesting no significant difference in their predictive capacities for in-hospital mortality. A meta-analysis by Peng et al. compared the prognostic assessment capabilities of the Child-Pugh and MELD scores across various clinical settings in liver cirrhosis [16]. These findings advocate for developing more refined prognostic tools tailored to specific cirrhotic complications. Bai et al. developed and validated a novel model named CAGIB for predicting the prognosis of patients with liver cirrhosis [17]. The CAGIB score, which had an AUC of 0.829 in the training cohort and 0.714 in the validation cohort, outperformed other prognostic models, such as Child-Pugh, MELD, MELD-Na, and NLR. The results proved the CAGIB score to be a strong predictor of in-hospital death.

Our research in cirrhosis has advanced diagnostics, management, and prognostication, emphasizing early detection and innovative treatments. We introduced the Liaoning scoring system for non-invasive diagnosis of EVs, highlighting the potential of CT to reduce reliance on invasive procedures. Our studies on PVT validate the efficacy of anticoagulation therapy, notably DOACs, in improving outcomes without increasing bleeding risks. Additionally, we explored prognostic assessment models, including the development of the CAGIB score, to better predict patient outcomes. This book aims to enhance patient care in cirrhosis through scientific collaboration and sharing knowledge globally, fostering advancements in the field.

Author details

Ran Wang*, Xiaozhong Guo and Xingshun Qi
Department of Gastroenterology, General Hospital of Northern Theater Command, Shenyang, China

*Address all correspondence to: wangran891017@163.com

References

[1] Devarbhavi H, Asrani SK, Arab JP, Nartey YA, Pose E, Kamath PS. Global burden of liver disease: 2023 update. Journal of Hepatology. 2023;**79**(2):516-537

[2] Garcia-Tsao G, Sanyal AJ, Grace ND, Carey W, Practice Guidelines Committee of the American Association for the Study of Liver D, Practice Parameters Committee of the American College of G. Prevention and management of gastroesophageal varices and variceal hemorrhage in cirrhosis. Hepatology. 2007;**46**(3):922-938

[3] Reverter E, Tandon P, Augustin S, et al. A MELD-based model to determine risk of mortality among patients with acute variceal bleeding. Gastroenterology. 2014;**146**(2):412-419 e413

[4] Jairath V, Rehal S, Logan R, et al. Acute variceal haemorrhage in the United Kingdom: Patient characteristics, management and outcomes in a nationwide audit. Digestive and Liver Disease. 2014;**46**(5):419-426

[5] Deng H, Qi X, Guo X. Diagnostic accuracy of APRI, AAR, FIB-4, FI, King, Lok, Forns, and FibroIndex scores in predicting the presence of esophageal varices in liver cirrhosis: A systematic review and meta-analysis. Medicine (Baltimore). 2015;**94**(42):e1795

[6] Qi X, Li Y, Wang R, et al. Liaoning score for prediction of esophageal varices in cirrhotic patients who had never undergone endoscopy: A Multicenter cross-sectional study in Liaoning Province, China. Advanced Therapy. 2019;**36**(8):2167-2178

[7] Li Q, Wu Y, Zhu Q, et al. External validation of Liaoning score for predicting esophageal varices in liver cirrhosis: A Chinese multicenter cross-sectional study. Annals of Translational Medicine. 2019;**7**(23):755

[8] Li Q, Wang R, Guo X, et al. Contrast-enhanced CT may Be a diagnostic alternative for gastroesophageal varices in cirrhosis with and without previous endoscopic variceal therapy. Gastroenterology Research and Practice. 2019;**2019**:6704673

[9] Nery F, Chevret S, Condat B, et al. Causes and consequences of portal vein thrombosis in 1,243 patients with cirrhosis: Results of a longitudinal study. Hepatology. 2015;**61**(2):660-667

[10] Qi X, Guo X, Yoshida EM, et al. Transient portal vein thrombosis in liver cirrhosis. BMC Medicine. 2018;**16**(1):83

[11] Wang L, Guo X, Xu X, et al. Anticoagulation favors thrombus recanalization and survival in patients with liver cirrhosis and portal vein thrombosis: Results of a meta-analysis. Advances in Therapy. 2021;**38**(1):495-520

[12] Li Z, Xu W, Wang L, et al. Risk of bleeding in liver cirrhosis receiving direct oral anticoagulants: A systematic review and meta-analysis. Thrombosis and Haemostasis. 2023;**123**(11):1072-1088

[13] Gao F, Wang L, Pan J, et al. Efficacy and safety of thrombolytic therapy for portal venous system thrombosis: A systematic review and meta-analysis. Journal of Internal Medicine. 2023;**293**(2):212-227

[14] Peng Y, Qi X, Tang S, et al. Child-Pugh, MELD, and ALBI scores for predicting the in-hospital mortality in cirrhotic patients with acute-on-chronic

liver failure. Expert Review of Gastroenterology & Hepatology. 2016;**10**(8):971-980

[15] Peng Y, Qi X, Dai J, Li H, Guo X. Child-Pugh versus MELD score for predicting the in-hospital mortality of acute upper gastrointestinal bleeding in liver cirrhosis. International Journal of Clinical and Experimental Medicine. 2015;**8**(1):751-757

[16] Peng Y, Qi X, Guo X. Child-Pugh versus MELD score for the assessment of prognosis in liver cirrhosis: A systematic review and meta-analysis of observational studies. Medicine (Baltimore). 2016;**95**(8):e2877

[17] Bai Z, Li B, Lin S, et al. Development and validation of CAGIB score for evaluating the prognosis of cirrhosis with acute gastrointestinal bleeding: A retrospective Multicenter Study. Advances in Therapy. 2019;**36**(11):3211-3220

Chapter 2

Noninvasive Diagnostic Methods in Liver Cirrhosis

Ying Peng, Shubei He and Ning Kang

Abstract

Liver cirrhosis is a condition characterized by the gradual development of liver fibrosis and the disruption of hepatic lobules. Patients who have decompensated cirrhosis face a significant risk of severe complications, including ascites, esophageal varices, liver failure, and hepatocellular carcinoma. Early diagnosis and timely intervention are crucial to preventing further liver damage, reducing morbidity and mortality associated with complications, and improving the prognosis. Additionally, timely diagnosis and accurate assessment of liver cirrhosis are critical for effective management and treatment. While liver biopsy has long been considered the gold standard for diagnosing cirrhosis, it has well-known limitations, including invasiveness, sampling error, and high expense. These limitations have restricted its widespread use in clinical practice. As a result, noninvasive diagnostic methods for liver cirrhosis have been proposed as alternatives to liver biopsy. Current noninvasive methods encompass liver and spleen stiffness measurements, ultrasound, computerized tomography, and magnetic resonance imaging, as well as serum biomarkers. Additionally, emerging technologies, such as omics, have led to the identification of novel biomarkers. However, the diagnostic performances of these methods vary among studies. Further, research and standardization of these methods are necessary to enhance their diagnostic accuracy and clinical utility in the evaluation of liver cirrhosis.

Keywords: liver stiffness measurement, spleen stiffness measurement, computerized tomography, serum biomarkers, noninvasive tests

1. Introduction

Liver cirrhosis is a pathology characterized by progressive hepatic fibrosis and lobular disruption [1]. Decompensated cirrhosis patients are at heightened risk of critical complications such as ascites, esophageal varices, hepatic failure, and hepatocellular carcinoma. Prompt diagnosis and intervention in liver cirrhosis, including its attendant complications, are paramount in mitigating further hepatic deterioration, decreasing associated morbidity and mortality, and thus enhancing patients' prognoses. Nevertheless, these imperatives face constraints in clinical application due to various limitations.

Liver biopsy has long been considered as the gold standard for diagnosing cirrhosis, whereas this method is beset with several potential limitations [2, 3]. Firstly, the biopsy sample's length may not accurately represent the liver's overall pathological state, with a longer biopsy sample potentially reducing the sampling error. It is generally accepted that a biopsy sample length of 15 mm suffices for stage assessment, though some reports advocate for a 25 mm length for more precise evaluation [3]. Additionally, a 16 gauge needle is deemed suitable for percutaneous liver biopsies. A second limitation involves variability in pathological assessments among pathologists, a challenge potentially mitigated by evaluation from specialized liver pathologists. Thirdly, liver biopsy, being invasive and costly, is unsuitable for widespread screening or longitudinal follow-up in the general population. Consequently, noninvasive diagnostic modalities have been proposed as pragmatic alternatives to liver biopsy, suitable for screening, monitoring, and follow-up. These encompass traditional techniques such as ultrasonography, computerized tomography, and magnetic resonance imaging, along with elastography for assessing liver and spleen stiffness, serum biomarkers and algorithm, and burgeoning methods including genetic models, omics, microbiome as well as artificial intelligence analyses.

2. Conventional imaging methods

Conventional imaging modalities, including abdominal ultrasonography, computerized tomography (CT), and magnetic resonance imaging (MRI), play significant roles in the diagnostic landscape of liver cirrhosis. Standard ultrasonography, notable for its convenience, cost-effectiveness, and lack of radiation exposure, is aptly suited for routine surveillance of liver cirrhosis and its complications, such as ascites, portal hypertension, and hepatocellular carcinoma (HCC). However, its reliance on operator expertise introduces subjectivity and interobserver variability. Additional confounding factors impacting its accuracy include abdominal air, obesity, and hepatic inflammation [4]. CT imaging, in contrast, surpasses ultrasonography in delineating morphological alterations of smaller hepatic lesions and in detecting complications such as varices, vascular changes, and liver nodules. Moreover, CT quantifies the total area of spontaneous portosystemic shunts, serving as a prognostic indicator for hepatic encephalopathy (HE) and mortality [5]. Nonetheless, its routine use is limited due to the associated radiation exposure. MRI holds a superior edge over both abdominal ultrasonography and CT in the detection of smaller nodules. However, its application is constrained by contraindications in patients with metal implants and by its relatively higher cost, limiting its routine usage. Additionally, these conventional methods are typically inadequate for the identification of early-stage liver cirrhosis, thus underscoring the need for more sensitive diagnostic tools [6].

3. Serum biomarkers and algorithms

Serum biomarkers, encompassing both direct and indirect indicators, play a pivotal role in the noninvasive assessment of liver fibrosis and cirrhosis (**Table 1**). Direct biomarkers are those constituents released into the bloodstream during fibrogenesis or remodeling of the extracellular matrix. This category includes hyaluronic acid, the N-terminal peptide of pro-collagen III, pro-collagen 3 neoepitope (PRO-C3), and tissue inhibitor of metalloproteinase 1, among others [7]. Notably, algorithms derived from these direct markers, such as the enhanced liver fibrosis (ELF) test, PRO-C3, FibroTest, and FibroMeter, have been formulated and patented. These tests are known for their ability to predict decompensation linked to advanced fibrosis (defined as

Serum biomarkers	Variables
Patented biomarkers	
FibroTest®	age, gender, α-2-macroglobulin, γGT, apolipoprotein A1, haptoglobin, total bilirubin
FibroMeter®	age, platelet count, prothrombin index, AST, α-2-macroglobulin, hyaluronate, urea
Flepascore®	bilirubin, γGT, hyaluronate, α-2-macroglobulin, age and gender
FibroSpectll®	α-2-macroglobulin, hyaluronate and TIMP-1
ELF®	age, hyaluronate, MMP-3 and TIMP-1
Non-patented biomarkers	
FIB-4	age (yr) × AST [U/L]/(platelets [10^9/L] × (ALT [U/L])1/2
APRI	AST (/ULN)/platelet (10^9/L) × 100
AAR	AST/ALT ratio
Forns Index	7.811–3.131 × ln(platelet count) + 0.781 × ln(GGT) + 3.467 × ln(age) - 0.014 × (cholesterol)
Fibroindex	1.738–0.064 × (platelets [10^4/mm^3]) + 0.005 × (AST [IU/L]) + 0.463 × (gamma globulin [g/dl])
Lok index	−5.56 - 0.0089 × platelet (10^3/mm^3) + 1.26 × AST/ALT ratio = 5.27 × INR
ADAPT	age, presence of diabetes, PRO-C3, and platelet count
NIS4	microRNA-34a-5p, α2-macroglobulins, YKL-40, HbA1c
	LSM, controlled attenuation parameter, AST
FibroScan-AST (FAST)	(−1.675 + 0.037 × age (yr) + 0.094 × BMI (kg/m^2) + 1.13 × IFG/diabetes (yes = 1, no = 0) + 0.99 × AST/ALT ratio - 0.013 × platelet count (×109/L) - 0.66 × albumin [g/dl])
NAFLD Fibrosis Score (NFS)	BMI ≥28 = 1; AST/ALT ratio ≥ 0.8 = 2; diabetes = 1; score ≥ 2,
BARD	
Emerging non-invasive tests based on serum biomarkers	
LSM-spleen diameter to platelet ratio score (LSPS)	LSM, spleen diameter, and platelet count
Agile 4/Agile 3+	LSM, platelet count, AAR, sex, diabetes

Abbreviation: AST, aspartate aminotransferase; ALT, alanine aminotransferase; TIMP-1, tissue inhibitor of metalloproteinases-1; GGT, gamma-glutamyl transferase; BMI, body mass index; IFG, impaired fasting glucose; MMP-3, matrix metalloproteinase-3; HbA1c, hemoglobin A1c; LSM, liver stiffness measurement; INR, international normalized ratio.

Table 1.
Noninvasive serum biomarkers in liver cirrhosis.

fibrosis stages 3 and 4). Conversely, indirect biomarkers typically reflect hepatocellular injury, inflammation, dysfunction, or portal hypertension [8]. Panels leveraging these indirect markers include fibrosis-4 index (FIB-4), aspartate aminotransferase-to-platelet ratio index (APRI) and aspartate aminotransferase-to-alanine aminotransferase ratio (AAR), Forns index, Lok index, or ADAPT. With the escalating global incidence of nonalcoholic fatty liver disease (NAFLD) worldwide, novel NITs have been proposed for the diagnosis of advanced fibrosis in these patients. The NAFLD fibrosis score (NFS), incorporating six elements, age, T2DM, BMI, AAR, albumin, and platelet count, has been developed from biopsy-proven NAFLD patients to identify liver fibrosis [9]. Additionally, the BARD score amalgamates AAR with BMI and the presence of T2DM. Its predictive value is constrained by the high prevalence of obesity and T2DM in the NAFLD cohort, leading to a majority of patients surpassing the defined threshold and resulting in a low positive predictive value (PPV) [10]. However, the diagnostic threshold of the NITs varies from different etiologies. For hepatitis B virus (HBV) or hepatitis C virus (HCV) infections, FIB-4 values below 1.45 and above 3.25 are interpreted as low and high stratification risks, respectively. In cases of NAFLD or alcohol-related liver disease (ALD), thresholds are set lower than

1.30 and higher than 2.67 for similar risk stratifications [11]. The accuracy of these serum biomarker panels in diagnostics is a subject of ongoing debate. Previous studies have indicated varying levels of efficacy, with some finding biomarkers, such as AAR predictive in certain contexts, such as chronic HCV infection, while others call for further validation and investigation, especially in diverse cohorts [12, 13]. In summary, while serum biomarker-based NITs exhibit high negative predictive values for excluding fibrosis or cirrhosis, their PPVs for diagnosis remain low, highlighting the need for continuous refinement and validation of these diagnostic tools [6].

4. Liver stiffness measurement (LSM) and spleen stiffness measurement (SSM)

Elastography methodologies have been advanced for LSM and SSM, encompassing techniques such as vibration-controlled transient elastography (VCTE), two-dimensional shear wave elastography (2D-SWE), point shear wave elastography (pSWE) (also named acoustic radiation force impulse imaging (ARFI)), and magnetic resonance elastography (MRE). The FibroScan® is capable of measuring stiffness values ranging from a minimum of 1.5 kPa to a maximum of 75.0 kPa. VCTE stands out for its convenience and cost-effectiveness in assessing fibrosis stages *via* LSM in patients. ARFI, in particular, offers insights into the relative structural stiffness of tissues juxtaposed with adjacent areas. This capacity to quantify absolute tissue modulus is pivotal for diverse clinical applications, facilitating the longitudinal monitoring of disease processes that manifest through tissue stiffening or softening, such as liver fibrosis and steatosis. Such capabilities are instrumental in determining the appropriate timing for initiating or ceasing treatment protocols and in staging disease progression and resolution [14]. Magnetic resonance elastography (MRE) has emerged as a significant advancement in this field [15, 16]. MRE's capability to estimate LSM and SSM enables the evaluation of portal hypertension in cirrhotic patients, though it does not directly correlate with hepatic venous pressure gradient (HVPG) response [17]. However, limitations of MRE include its cost, time-intensive nature, infeasibility as a bedside procedure, and inapplicability in the presence of metal implants.

Baveno VI consensus recommended compensated advanced chronic liver disease (cACLD) patients with LSM < 40 kPa, and platelet count >150,000/μl could be waived from esophagogastroduodenoscopy (EGD). However, meta-analysis has indicated that the Baveno VI criteria, with a pooled sensitivity of 0.97 and specificity of 0.32, might misclassify high-risk varices (HRVs) [18]. To improve diagnostic accuracy, the Expanded Baveno VI criteria were proposed, which include a platelet count $>110 \times 10^9$ cells/μL and a TE < 25 kPa, potentially avoiding unnecessary EGD [19]. A recent study indicated that Baveno VI and Baveno VII criteria are not accurate for screening HRVs and CSPH in patients with HCC [20].

For patients with liver cirrhosis who develop clinically significant portal hypertension (CSPH), there is an elevated risk of decompensated events and liver-related mortality. The current gold standard for diagnosing CSPH is HVPG measurement [21]. LSM and SSM are valuable noninvasive alternatives for detecting and monitoring CSPH, correlating well with HVPG. LSM values >20–25 kPa and SSM values >40–45 kPa indicate a high likelihood of CSPH [22]. In a prospective study, Foucher et al. asserted the efficacy of LSM for diagnosing cirrhosis and its complications such as esophageal varices, HCC, and ascites in patients with chronic liver diseases, with values ranging from 12.5 to 75.5 kPa [23]. SSM serves as a direct and dynamic proxy for portal pressure, offering the potential to monitor the severity and improvement of portal hypertension and act as a surrogate marker for clinical outcomes. Notably, SSM appears more effective than LSM in monitoring treatment response in clinical trials aimed at reducing portal hypertension. The Baveno VII consensus recommended that an SSM $\leq$ 40 kPa could obviate the need for numerous unnecessary EGDs while also decreasing the incidence of diagnostic errors [22]. It has been reported that integrating SSM with the Baveno VI criteria resulted in increased specificity for excluding HRVs in HBV-related cirrhosis patients undergoing antiviral therapy [24]. Another research confirmed the efficacy of SSM in diagnosing CSPH and demonstrated that incorporating SSM could enhance the accuracy of the Baveno VII criteria in patients with metabolic-associated fatty liver disease (NAFLD) [25]. A meta-analysis showed that SSM in combination with Baveno VII can reduce the diagnostic gray zone for CSPH [26].

In clinical practice, the availability of NITs may guide patient evaluation approaches. LSM and SSM assessments using 2D-SWE have shown promising results for diagnosing cirrhosis in patients with autoimmune hepatitis, potentially less influenced by inflammation [27]. A single-center study from Japan indicated that SSM *via* ARFI can moderately accurately predict mortality in cirrhotic patients [28].

5. Emerging technologies

5.1 Imaging-based technologies

Recent advancements in imaging-based methodologies have emerged for the diagnosis of liver fibrosis and cirrhosis, leveraging ultrasonography, CT, MRI, and elastography. A noninvasive approach involving platelet count and spleen diameter has been proposed for predicting esophageal varices in patients with cirrhosis [29]. Subsequent research endeavors have sought to validate its effectiveness in both detecting and excluding esophageal varices, regardless of the underlying cause and severity of liver cirrhosis [30, 31]. Additionally, cutting-edge three-dimensional technologies are being explored. A noteworthy prospective head-to-head study by Loomba et al. demonstrated that 3D magnetic resonance elastography (3D-MRE) significantly outperforms its 2D counterpart in diagnosing advanced fibrosis, evidenced by an impressive AUC of 0.981 [32]. Despite its diagnostic superiority, the cost-effectiveness of 3D-MRE warrants further exploration to assess its viability for widespread clinical application. A novel ultrasound-based approach, three-dimensional multi-frequency shear wave absolute vibro-elastography (3D S-WAVE) with a matrix array, has been introduced. This technique has shown diagnostic capabilities comparable to MRE for liver fibrosis but offers advantages in terms of accessibility and cost. This innovation makes advanced diagnostic technology potentially available to a broader patient demographic, bridging the gap between high end, costly diagnostics and the practical needs of diverse healthcare settings [33]. Based on LSM, Kim et al. proposed a novel noninvasive model, the LSM-spleen diameter to platelet ratio score (LSPS), for predicting HRVs in HBV-related liver cirrhosis [34]. The variceal risk index (VRI), consisting of LSM, spleen diameter, and platelet count, has been effective in identifying CSPH and HRVs in patients with biopsy-proven compensated cirrhosis [35]. In a multicenter study, Sanyal et al. developed two novel scores, Agile 4 and Agile 3+, combining LSM with laboratory and demographic data to diagnose cirrhosis in NAFLD patients, demonstrating superior diagnostic capabilities compared to FIB-4 and LSM alone [36]. Another study also confirmed the superiority of Agile 3+ for the prediction of disease severity and liver-related events in NAFLD [37]. Several studies have compared the diagnostic capabilities of noninvasive models in chronic liver diseases, but the results remain controversial. A comparative analysis showed that a model combining LSM with SSM was more effective than other noninvasive models (LSPS, VRI, AAR, and Baveno VI criteria) in predicting HRVs in patients with viral cirrhosis [38]. Cho et al. assessed the diagnostic and prognostic values of various noninvasive fibrosis markers in patients with alcohol-related cirrhosis. Their findings indicated that LSM and LSPS outperformed other noninvasive fibrosis indices in predicting CSPH in patients with compensated cirrhosis [39]. However, the study by Colecchia et al. revealed that SSM was a valuable noninvasive tool for assessing varying degrees of portal hypertension and esophageal varices in HCV-related cirrhotic patients, outperforming the platelet count/spleen diameter and LSPS [40]. Notably, the Lok index was uniquely effective in enhancing the predictive accuracy of the model for end-stage liver disease (MELD) score for overall mortality in decompensated cirrhosis cases [39]. The LiverRisk score, which comprised age, sex, fasting glucose, cholesterol, AST, ALT, GGT, and platelet count, could predict liver fibrosis and liver-related outcomes in the general population [41].

5.2 Genetic prediction models

Prior research has suggested the potential application of gene signatures in the risk stratification for liver cirrhosis, particularly in chronic HBV and HCV [42, 43]. These studies have indicated that specific genetic markers could be instrumental in categorizing the risk levels associated with liver cirrhosis. One notable finding is the role of dynamic changes in the DNA methylation of the peroxisome proliferator-activated receptor gamma (PPARγ) in fibrogenesis. Such alterations in methylation patterns could serve as a promising biomarker for stratifying the risk of fibrosis progression in NAFLD [44]. Furthermore, the prevalence of a missense variant in the patatin-like phospholipase domain-containing protein 3 (PNPLA3), specifically the p.I148M variant, is significant (>20%) in the global population. This genetic variation has been associated with an increased risk of steatosis, cirrhosis, and HCC across various etiologies, emphasizing the genetic predisposition to these liver conditions [45]. Genetic risk scores, which amalgamate multiple risk polymorphisms, present a promising tool for identifying individuals predisposed to cirrhosis from an early age. A recent study incorporating 12 genetic risk alleles found that patients in the highest 20% bracket of polygenic risk were more than twice as likely to develop cirrhosis compared to those in the lowest 20% risk group. This finding underscores the potential of polygenic risk scores to quantify an individual's comprehensive genetic risk for cirrhosis [46]. The integration of polygenic risk scores, encompassing hundreds or thousands of genetic risk alleles, represents a significant advance in understanding the complex genetic underpinnings of liver cirrhosis [47]. This approach aims to provide a holistic assessment of an individual's genetic predisposition to cirrhosis, offering valuable insights for both preventive strategies and personalized medical interventions.

6. Microbiome

The alterations in the diversity and composition of the gut microbiome and its derivatives are increasingly recognized as crucial factors in the initiation and progression of liver diseases [48, 49]. In an innovative approach, Loomba et al. employed whole-genome shotgun sequencing of DNA from fecal samples, coupled with random forest analysis, to develop a predictive model. This model effectively identifies advanced fibrosis in patients with NAFLD, signifying a significant leap in noninvasive liver disease diagnostics [50]. Furthermore, the analysis of gut microbiome signatures has yielded promising results in the prediction of liver cirrhosis. These microbiome-based models exhibit considerable accuracy, underscoring the potential of gut microbiota as a biomarker for liver health and disease [51]. This emerging field, bridging gastroenterology and hepatology, opens new avenues for early detection and intervention strategies in liver cirrhosis, leveraging the intricate interplay between the gut microbiome and liver function.

6.1 Omics and artificial intelligence

The utilization of a combined noninvasive serum protein signature, employing SomaScan® technology, has demonstrated proficiency in accurately predicting HVPG response in HCV liver cirrhosis post-sustained virological response (SVR) [52]. Additionally, the serum caspase-cleaved fragment of keratin-18 has been identified as a marker correlated with the histological severity and liver-related mortality, not only in alcohol-related liver disease but also in NAFLD [53, 54]. Recent advancements in the field have seen the integration of mass spectrometry (MS)-based proteomics with machine learning (ML) methodologies to effectively detect significant fibrosis, showcasing robust performance [55]. In a pioneering study by Corey et al., the application of aptamer-based proteomics technology revealed that the ADAMTSL2 protein could serve as a biomarker for identifying individuals at risk of nonalcoholic steatohepatitis and fibrosis [56]. Additionally, a convolutional neural network model based on trichrome-stained liver biopsy slides has been developed to predict CSPH in patients with biopsy-proven NASH cirrhosis [57]. Another recent advancement involves an ML model based on histologic features, capable of accurately predicting HVPG, CSPH, the development of varices, and changes in HVPG in NASH cirrhosis [58]. Liu et al. innovatively utilized ML to accurately extract liver capsule features from high-frequency ultrasound images, aiding in the diagnosis of cirrhosis [59]. ML models performed better overall than FibroScan, FIB-4, FAST, and NFS. ML could be an effective tool for identifying clinically significant liver fibrosis and cirrhosis in patients with NAFLD. A recent study showed that LSM combined with an ML model could accurately identify MASLD-related cirrhosis and advanced fibrosis [60].

In conclusion, noninvasive tests offer a more affordable, convenient, and safer alternative for screening and monitoring liver conditions compared to liver biopsy. The accumulating body of evidence supports their efficacy in facilitating informed clinical decision-making. However, it is noteworthy that the diagnostic performance of these noninvasive tests exhibits variability across different studies. To optimize their diagnostic accuracy and clinical utility in assessing liver cirrhosis, further well-designed multicenter research studies for the validation of these methodologies are imperative.

Author details

Ying Peng[1*], Shubei He[1] and Ning Kang[2]

1 Department of Gastroenterology, the First Affiliated Hospital (Southwest Hospital) to Third Military Medical University (Army Medical University), Chongqing, China

2 Department of Gastroenterology, The First People's Hospital of Chongqing Liangjiang New Area, Chongqing, China

*Address all correspondence to: ying.peng@cldcsw.org

References

[1] Gines P, Krag A, Abraldes JG, et al. Liver cirrhosis. Lancet. 2021;**398**(10308):1359-1376

[2] Davison BA, Harrison SA, Cotter G, et al. Suboptimal reliability of liver biopsy evaluation has implications for randomized clinical trials. Journal of Hepatology. 2020;**73**(6):1322-1332

[3] Bedossa P, Dargere D, Paradis V. Sampling variability of liver fibrosis in chronic hepatitis C. Hepatology. 2003;**38**(6):1449-1457

[4] Trinchet JC, Chaffaut C, Bourcier V, et al. Ultrasonographic surveillance of hepatocellular carcinoma in cirrhosis: A randomized trial comparing 3- and 6-month periodicities. Hepatology. 2011;**54**(6):1987-1997

[5] Praktiknjo M, Simon-Talero M, Romer J, et al. Total area of spontaneous portosystemic shunts independently predicts hepatic encephalopathy and mortality in liver cirrhosis. Journal of Hepatology. 2020;**72**(6):1140-1150

[6] European Association for the Study of the Liver. Electronic address eee, Clinical Practice Guideline P, Chair, et al. EASL clinical practice guidelines on non-invasive tests for evaluation of liver disease severity and prognosis - 2021 update. Journal of Hepatology. 2021;**75**(3):659-689

[7] Leeming DJ, Karsdal MA, Byrjalsen I, et al. Novel serological neo-epitope markers of extracellular matrix proteins for the detection of portal hypertension. Alimentary Pharmacology & Therapeutics. 2013;**38**(9):1086-1096

[8] Lindvig KP, Hansen TL, Madsen BS, et al. Diagnostic accuracy of routine liver function tests to identify patients with significant and advanced alcohol-related liver fibrosis. Scandinavian Journal of Gastroenterology. 2021;**56**(9):1088-1095

[9] Angulo P, Hui JM, Marchesini G, et al. The NAFLD fibrosis score: A noninvasive system that identifies liver fibrosis in patients with NAFLD. Hepatology. 2007;**45**(4):846-854

[10] McPherson S, Stewart SF, Henderson E, et al. Simple non-invasive fibrosis scoring systems can reliably exclude advanced fibrosis in patients with non-alcoholic fatty liver disease. Gut. 2010;**59**(9):1265-1269

[11] Anstee QM, Lawitz EJ, Alkhouri N, et al. Noninvasive tests accurately identify advanced fibrosis due to NASH: Baseline data from the STELLAR trials. Hepatology. 2019;**70**(5):1521-1530

[12] Sheth SG, Flamm SL, Gordon FD, et al. AST/ALT ratio predicts cirrhosis in patients with chronic hepatitis C virus infection. The American Journal of Gastroenterology. 1998;**93**(1):44-48

[13] Imperiale TF, Said AT, Cummings OW, et al. Need for validation of clinical decision aids: Use of the AST/ALT ratio in predicting cirrhosis in chronic hepatitis C. The American Journal of Gastroenterology. 2000;**95**(9):2328-2332

[14] Nightingale K, Palmeri M, Trahey G. Analysis of contrast in images generated with transient acoustic radiation force. Ultrasound in Medicine & Biology. 2006;**32**(1):61-72

[15] Muthupillai R, Lomas DJ, Rossman PJ, et al. Magnetic resonance elastography by direct visualization

of propagating acoustic strain waves. Science. 1995;**269**(5232):1854-1857

[16] Rouviere O, Yin M, Dresner MA, et al. MR elastography of the liver: Preliminary results. Radiology. 2006;**240**(2):440-448

[17] Danielsen KV, Hove JD, Nabilou P, et al. Using MR elastography to assess portal hypertension and response to beta-blockers in patients with cirrhosis. Liver International. 2021;**41**(9):2149-2158

[18] Stafylidou M, Paschos P, Katsoula A, et al. Performance of Baveno VI and expanded Baveno VI criteria for excluding high-risk varices in patients with chronic liver diseases: A systematic review and meta-analysis. Clinical Gastroenterology and Hepatology. 2019;**17**(9):1744-1755, e1711

[19] Augustin S, Pons M, Maurice JB, et al. Expanding the Baveno VI criteria for the screening of varices in patients with compensated advanced chronic liver disease. Hepatology. 2017;**66**(6):1980-1988

[20] Allaire M, Campion B, Demory A, et al. Baveno VI and VII criteria are not suitable for screening for large varices or clinically significant portal hypertension in patients with hepatocellular carcinoma. Alimentary Pharmacology & Therapeutics. 2023;**58**(3):346-356

[21] de Franchis R, Baveno VIF. Expanding consensus in portal hypertension: Report of the Baveno VI consensus workshop: Stratifying risk and individualizing care for portal hypertension. Journal of Hepatology. 2015;**63**(3):743-752

[22] de Franchis R, Bosch J, Garcia-Tsao G, et al. Baveno VII - renewing consensus in portal hypertension. Journal of Hepatology. 2022;**76**(4):959-974

[23] Foucher J, Chanteloup E, Vergniol J, et al. Diagnosis of cirrhosis by transient elastography (FibroScan): A prospective study. Gut. 2006;**55**(3):403-408

[24] Wang H, Wen B, Chang X, et al. Baveno VI criteria and spleen stiffness measurement rule out high-risk varices in virally suppressed HBV-related cirrhosis. Journal of Hepatology. 2021;**74**(3):584-592

[25] Odriozola A, Puente A, Cuadrado A, et al. High accuracy of spleen stiffness measurement in diagnosing clinically significant portal hypertension in metabolic-associated fatty liver disease. Liver International. 2023;**43**(7):1446-1457

[26] Dajti E, Ravaioli F, Zykus R, et al. Accuracy of spleen stiffness measurement for the diagnosis of clinically significant portal hypertension in patients with compensated advanced chronic liver disease: A systematic review and individual patient data meta-analysis. The Lancet Gastroenterology & Hepatology. 2023;**8**(9):816-828

[27] Janik MK, Kruk B, Szczepankiewicz B, et al. Measurement of liver and spleen stiffness as complementary methods for assessment of liver fibrosis in autoimmune hepatitis. Liver International. 2021;**41**(2):348-356

[28] Takuma Y, Morimoto Y, Takabatake H, et al. Measurement of spleen stiffness with acoustic radiation force impulse imaging predicts mortality and hepatic decompensation in patients with liver cirrhosis. Clinical Gastroenterology and Hepatology. 2017;**15**(11):1782-1790, e1784

[29] Giannini E, Botta F, Borro P, et al. Platelet count/spleen diameter ratio: Proposal and validation of a non-invasive parameter to predict the presence of

oesophageal varices in patients with liver cirrhosis. Gut. 2003;**52**(8):1200-1205

[30] Giannini EG, Zaman A, Kreil A, et al. Platelet count/spleen diameter ratio for the noninvasive diagnosis of esophageal varices: Results of a multicenter, prospective, validation study. The American Journal of Gastroenterology. 2006;**101**(11):2511-2519

[31] Giannini EG, Botta F, Borro P, et al. Application of the platelet count/spleen diameter ratio to rule out the presence of oesophageal varices in patients with cirrhosis: A validation study based on follow-up. Digestive and Liver Disease. 2005;**37**(10):779-785

[32] Loomba R, Cui J, Wolfson T, et al. Novel 3D magnetic resonance elastography for the noninvasive diagnosis of advanced fibrosis in NAFLD: A prospective study. The American Journal of Gastroenterology. 2016;**111**(7):986-994

[33] Zeng Q, Honarvar M, Schneider C, et al. Three-dimensional multi-frequency shear wave absolute vibro-elastography (3D S-WAVE) with a matrix array transducer: Implementation and preliminary In vivo study of the liver. IEEE Transactions on Medical Imaging. 2021;**40**(2):648-660

[34] Kim BK, Han KH, Park JY, et al. A liver stiffness measurement-based, noninvasive prediction model for high-risk esophageal varices in B-viral liver cirrhosis. The American Journal of Gastroenterology. 2010;**105**(6):1382-1390

[35] Berzigotti A, Seijo S, Arena U, et al. Elastography, spleen size, and platelet count identify portal hypertension in patients with compensated cirrhosis. Gastroenterology. 2013;**144**(1):102-111, e101

[36] Sanyal AJ, Foucquier J, Younossi ZM, et al. Enhanced diagnosis of advanced fibrosis and cirrhosis in individuals with NAFLD using FibroScan-based agile scores. Journal of Hepatology. 2023;**78**(2):247-259

[37] Pennisi G, Enea M, Pandolfo A, et al. AGILE 3+ score for the diagnosis of advanced fibrosis and for predicting liver-related events in NAFLD. Clinical Gastroenterology and Hepatology. 2023;**21**(5):1293-1302, e1295

[38] Yang LB, Gao X, Li H, et al. Non-invasive model for predicting high-risk esophageal varices based on liver and spleen stiffness. World Journal of Gastroenterology. 2023;**29**(25):4072-4084

[39] Cho EJ, Kim MY, Lee JH, et al. Diagnostic and prognostic values of noninvasive predictors of portal hypertension in patients with alcoholic cirrhosis. PLoS One. 2015;**10**(7):e0133935

[40] Colecchia A, Montrone L, Scaioli E, et al. Measurement of spleen stiffness to evaluate portal hypertension and the presence of esophageal varices in patients with HCV-related cirrhosis. Gastroenterology. 2012;**143**(3):646-654

[41] Serra-Burriel M, Juanola A, Serra-Burriel F, et al. Development, validation, and prognostic evaluation of a risk score for long-term liver-related outcomes in the general population: A multicohort study. Lancet. 2023;**402**(10406):988-996

[42] Huang H, Shiffman ML, Friedman S, et al. A 7 gene signature identifies the risk of developing cirrhosis in patients with chronic hepatitis C. Hepatology. 2007;**46**(2):297-306

[43] Xu MY, Qu Y, Li Z, et al. A 6 gene signature identifies the risk of developing

cirrhosis in patients with chronic hepatitis B. Frontiers in Bioscience (Landmark Ed). 2016;**21**(3):479-486

[44] Hardy T, Zeybel M, Day CP, et al. Plasma DNA methylation: A potential biomarker for stratification of liver fibrosis in non-alcoholic fatty liver disease. Gut. 2017;**66**(7):1321-1328

[45] Gellert-Kristensen H, Richardson TG, Davey Smith G, et al. Combined effect of PNPLA3, TM6SF2, and HSD17B13 variants on risk of cirrhosis and hepatocellular carcinoma in the general population. Hepatology. 2020;**72**(3):845-856

[46] Emdin CA, Haas M, Ajmera V, et al. Association of genetic variation with cirrhosis: A multi-trait genome-wide association and gene-environment interaction study. Gastroenterology. 2021;**160**(5):1620-1633, e1613

[47] Torkamani A, Wineinger NE, Topol EJ. The personal and clinical utility of polygenic risk scores. Nature Reviews. Genetics. 2018;**19**(9):581-590

[48] Tilg H, Cani PD, Mayer EA. Gut microbiome and liver diseases. Gut. 2016;**65**(12):2035-2044

[49] Qin N, Yang F, Li A, et al. Alterations of the human gut microbiome in liver cirrhosis. Nature. 2014;**513**(7516):59-64

[50] Loomba R, Seguritan V, Li W, et al. Gut microbiome-based metagenomic signature for non-invasive detection of advanced fibrosis in human nonalcoholic fatty liver disease. Cell Metabolism. 2017;**25**(5):1054-1062, e1055

[51] Oh TG, Kim SM, Caussy C, et al. A universal gut-microbiome-derived signature predicts cirrhosis. Cell Metabolism. 2020;**32**(5):901

[52] Richards SM, Guo F, Zou H, et al. Non-invasive candidate protein signature predicts hepatic venous pressure gradient reduction in cirrhotic patients after sustained virologic response. Liver International. 2023;**43**(9):1984-1994

[53] Mueller S, Nahon P, Rausch V, et al. Caspase-cleaved keratin-18 fragments increase during alcohol withdrawal and predict liver-related death in patients with alcoholic liver disease. Hepatology. 2017;**66**(1):96-107

[54] Atkinson SR, Grove JI, Liebig S, et al. In severe alcoholic hepatitis, serum keratin-18 fragments are diagnostic, prognostic, and theragnostic biomarkers. The American Journal of Gastroenterology. 2020;**115**(11):1857-1868

[55] Niu L, Thiele M, Geyer PE, et al. Noninvasive proteomic biomarkers for alcohol-related liver disease. Nature Medicine. 2022;**28**(6):1277-1287

[56] Corey KE, Pitts R, Lai M, et al. ADAMTSL2 protein and a soluble biomarker signature identify at-risk non-alcoholic steatohepatitis and fibrosis in adults with NAFLD. Journal of Hepatology. 2022;**76**(1):25-33

[57] Bosch J, Chung C, Carrasco-Zevallos OM, et al. A machine learning approach to liver histological evaluation predicts clinically significant portal hypertension in NASH cirrhosis. Hepatology. 2021;**74**(6):3146-3160

[58] Noureddin M, Goodman Z, Tai D, et al. Machine learning liver histology scores correlate with portal hypertension assessments in nonalcoholic steatohepatitis cirrhosis. Alimentary Pharmacology & Therapeutics. 2023;**57**(4):409-417

[59] Liu Y, Liu X, Wang S, et al. A novel method for accurate extraction of liver

capsule and auxiliary diagnosis of liver cirrhosis based on high-frequency ultrasound images. Computers in Biology and Medicine. 2020;**125**:104002

[60] Fan R, Yu N, Li G, et al. Machine-learning model comprising five clinical indices and liver stiffness measurement can accurately identify MASLD-related liver fibrosis. Liver International. 2024;**44**(3):749-759

Chapter 3

Non-Selective Beta-Blockers in Patients with Cirrhosis: Current Evidence and Controversy

Ting Wang, Cai'e Wang, Hongyu Li and Ran Wang

Abstract

Non-selective beta-blockers (NSBBs) are the cornerstone of management of liver cirrhosis and its complications. They decrease portal vein blood flow and portal vein pressure via antagonism of β_1 and β_2 receptors, thereby improving the hyperdynamic circulatory status and reducing the risk of decompensated events in cirrhotic patients with portal hypertension (PH). Currently, NSBBs have been recommended for the primary and secondary prevention of variceal bleeding in patients with cirrhosis. Nevertheless, it has been noted that the clinical risk-benefit ratio appears to deteriorate for NSBBs in patients with advanced liver cirrhosis. Considering that the use of NSBBs in the clinical practice of cirrhotic patients remains controversial, this chapter aims to summarize the evidence of current recommendations and controversies regarding the use of NSBBs in patients with cirrhosis.

Keywords: liver cirrhosis, NSBBs, PH, varices, ascites, spontaneous bacterial peritonitis, renal dysfunction, portal vein thrombosis

1. Introduction

Liver cirrhosis, characterized by progressive fibrosis and liver injury, is the end stage of several liver diseases [1]. Portal hypertension (PH), a primary consequence of cirrhosis, may cause serious complications, including variceal bleeding (VB), ascites, and hepatic encephalopathy (HE) [2, 3]. Currently, hepatic venous pressure gradient (HVPG) measurement is considered the gold standard test for the diagnosis of PH in clinical practice [4]. HVPG represents the actual liver portal perfusion pressure, and its value greater than 5 mmHg indicates PH. Portal pressure increases with progressive disease, ultimately surpassing cut-off values of 10 mmHg, which marks the occurrence of clinically significant PH (CSPH). Patients with CSPH and cirrhosis exhibit splanchnic and peripheral vasodilatation, resulting in increased heart rate and cardiac output, which is characteristic of the hyperdynamic circulation state of advanced PH [5, 6].

Non-selective beta-blockers (NSBBs) are the cornerstone of management of PH [7]. NSBBs reduce peripheral blood flow via antagonism of β_1 receptor, thereby reducing the heart rate and cardiac output, as well as splanchnic vasoconstriction

IntechOpen

through inhibition of β_2 receptor, thereby decreasing portal venous blood flow and portal pressure [8, 9]. Accordingly, NSBBs could improve the hyperdynamic circulatory status of CSPH patients and decrease the development of decompensated events in patients with compensated cirrhosis. Additionally, NSBBs may reduce bacterial translocation and inflammatory responses through non-hemodynamic mechanisms [10]. The traditional NSBBs commonly used in clinical practice include propranolol, nadolol, and timolol. Carvedilol is a novel NSBBs with an intrinsic anti-α-adrenergic activity, which stimulates the release of nitric oxide and causes intrahepatic vasodilatation, thereby further decreasing portal pressure [11].

According to the updated consensus and guidelines, NSBBs are specifically recommended for primary or secondary prophylaxis of VB in patients with high-risk varices [12–14]. It has been recently shown that NSBBs are not always beneficial to all cirrhotic patients [15]. Tonon et al. identified that the use of NSBBs may increase the risk of acute decompensation and non-acute decompensation in compensated patients [16]. In the window hypothesis, as proposed by Krag et al., it was suggested that the efficacy and safety of NSBBs may vary based on the spectrum of cirrhosis [17]. They questioned the use of NSBBs in early cirrhosis, which is free of medium or large varices, and warned to avoid NSBBs in patients with advanced cirrhosis and refractory ascites. This chapter aims to summarize the existing evidence on the indications and controversies for NSBBs in patients with cirrhosis, in order to provide a reference for the use of NSBBs in the clinical practice.

2. NSBBs in cirrhosis: indications

2.1 Clinically significant portal hypertension

CSPH is defined as HVPG ≥10 mmHg, as decompensation may develop after achieving this threshold [18]. Indeed, CSPH is the strong predictor of PH-associated complications such as VB, ascites, and HE in patients with compensated cirrhosis [19]. NSBB-induced reduction of HVPG at least 10% from baseline may prevent the first episode of VB and ascites [12]. A randomized, double-blind, multicenter trial (PREDESCI) in Spain included 201 compensated cirrhotic patients with CSPH and without high-risk varices. Patients were randomized to treatment with placebo or NSBBs (propranolol or carvedilol depending on hemodynamic response). Hemodynamic response to NSBBs was determined as a decrease of HVPG of ≥10% after 20 minutes of intravenous propranolol (0.15 mg/kg). They found that primary outcomes such as ascites, VB, or HE occurred in 16% of patients in the NSBBs group vs. 27% in the placebo group ($P = 0.041$). The difference was due to a reduced incidence of ascites ($P = 0{\cdot}0297$) [20]. An individual participant data meta-analysis of four randomized controlled trials (RCTs) revealed that the risk of decompensation in the carvedilol group was significantly lower than in the control group, which included endoscopic variceal ligation (EVL) and placebo among compensated patients with CSPH ($P = 0.017$) [21]. Kumar et al. randomly assigned 136 acute-on-chronic liver failure patients who were definitively diagnosed with CSPH and had no or small varices to carvedilol or placebo groups, which demonstrated that the use of carvedilol improved 28-day survival and reduced the risk of acute kidney injury (AKI) [22]. Thus, it appears to suggest that patients may benefit from the initiation of NSBBs once the CSPH has been diagnosed, whatever the status of the varices.

Notably, it is suggested that carvedilol is more effective in decreasing HVPG than propranolol or nadolol, including propranolol non-responders, with about 75% of patients achieving an HVPG response [23]. Besides, the Baveno VII consensus indicated that administration with NSBBs should be considered to prevent decompensation in patients with CSPH. Carvedilol is recommended as the preferred NSBBs for compensated cirrhosis compared to the traditional NSBBs (i.e., propranolol and nadolol) [12]. Overall, screening patients with CSPH in compensation cirrhosis for prompt initiation of NSBBs (preferred to carvedilol) may improve prognosis.

2.2 Primary prophylaxis

Currently, international guidelines suggest that NSBBs and EVL are similarly effective for primary prophylaxis, which are both recommended for patients with high-risk varices such as medium to large varices or small varices with red signs or Child-Pugh C [12, 13].

In a study by McDowell et al., 152 patients were included to evaluate the efficacy of carvedilol for the primary prevention of VB and survival. It showed that the median survival was significantly higher in the carvedilol group than in the EVL group (7.8 vs. 4.2 years, P = 0.03) [24]. A meta-analysis of 32 RCTs showed that monotherapy with NSBBs may reduce the risk of the first VB and mortality in cirrhotic patients with large varices, with a lower incidence of serious complications than EVL [25]. However, both these studies included patients with compensated cirrhosis and those with decompensated cirrhosis. Notably, the hemodynamic response of patients to NSBBs in cirrhosis varies across the spectrum of cirrhosis [26, 27]. In addition, the primary management goals for patients with cirrhosis also depend on the stage of cirrhosis. In patients with compensated cirrhosis, the major objective of treatment is not limited to the prevention of VB, which must focus on the prevention of decompensation events (ascites and HE). Thus, it is now preferred to choose treatments based on the stage of the disease. A competing-risk meta-analysis of 11 RCTs evaluated the efficacy of NSBBs vs. EVL on survival in patients with high-risk varices, stratifying risk based on the compensated/decompensated stage of cirrhosis. It showed that treatment with NSBBs had significantly improved survival compared with EVL in compensated cirrhotic patients, but in patients with decompensated cirrhosis, the survival was similar between the two therapies [28].

It is worth noting that the development of adverse events and the economic costs should be also considered while effective treatments are selected. Treatment with NSBBs has a lower risk of serious complications such as esophageal ulcers and esophageal perforation compared to EVL, which is more easily obtained, less depending on specialized endoscopic equipment like EVL, and has a higher economic efficiency.

2.3 Secondary prophylaxis

Nowadays, updated international guidelines and consensus recommend the use of NSBBs combined with EVL for secondary prophylaxis of VB [12, 13]. In addition, a combination therapy of NSBBs and isosorbide-mononitrate (IsMn) is also recommended as secondary prophylaxis of VB by the Japanese Society of Gastroenterology [14]. Kong et al. included 43 RCTs to compare the efficacy of medications, endoscopic options, transjugular intrahepatic portosystemic shunts (TIPS), and mainstay combination therapies in cirrhotic patients with at least one episode VB. It showed that nadolol combined with ISMN may be a preferable option to reduce mortality associated with rebleeding in patients with cirrhosis [29]. Another network meta-analysis of 26 RCTs showed that nadolol combined with EVL may be the preferred option for preventing rebleeding in cirrhotic patients who had one previous episode of VB, while NSBBs combined with ISMN may be potential alternatives to improve mortality [30]. Moreover, Jachs et al. identified that the cumulative incidences of rebleeding (P = 0.027) and liver-related death (P = 0.036) were significantly lower in patients administered with carvedilol combined with EVL versus propranolol combined with EVL [31].

3. NSBBs in cirrhosis: controversies

3.1 Preprimary prophylaxis

Currently, there is inadequate evidence to support the use of NSBBs for the prevention of the development or growth of varices in cirrhotic patients with no varices. Groszmann et al. randomly assigned 213 patients with HVPG ≥6 mm Hg without varices to the timolol group and the placebo group. During a median follow-up of 54.9 months, the incidence of the primary endpoint (development of gastroesophageal varices or VB) was not significantly different between the timolol and the placebo groups (39 vs. 40%, P = 0.89). Besides, severe adverse events were reported with a higher proportion of patients in the timolol group compared with the placebo group (18 vs. 6%, P = 0.006) [32]. It's worth noting that most patients (59%) without varices had only subclinical PH (SPH) in this study. However, NSBBs exert a stronger effect for reduction of portal pressure in CSPH patients than in SPH patients who do not develop increased cardiac output and hyperdynamic circulation, which is a prerequisite for NSBBs to exert their activity [26]. This explains why NSBBs are ineffective generally in preprimary prophylaxis. Similarly, a meta-analysis of six RCTs including patients with no or small varices also showed no significant benefit of NSBBs compared with placebo for the prevention of large varices, first VB, and death [33].

In contrast, Bhardwaj et al. showed that a lower proportion of patients in the carvedilol group had a progression of small varices to large varices compared to the placebo group [34]. Di Pascoli et al. conducted a long-term observation of patients who started with NSBBs when diagnosed with small varices versus those treated with NSBBs after the confirmation of large varices by endoscopy. They also found that the small-varices group had a significantly lower rate of adverse outcomes (progression of varices or VB or death) than the large-varices group and had lower economic costs [35]. In general, the evidence is conflicting regarding the effect of NSBBs on slowing the development of small varices into large varices in cirrhotic patients. Thus, treatment should be focused on elimination or control of the cause in liver disease at this stage. Additionally, it is also important to monitor the magnitude of hemodynamic changes to determine a hyperdynamic circulatory state and prevent decompensated events in patients with no or small varices.

3.2 Ascites and refractory ascites

In 2010, a milestone study by Serste et al. revealed that treatment with propranolol was associated with poor survival in patients with refractory ascites. This study created a lively debate in the hepatology field [36]. Notably, the NSBBs group had a higher proportion of Child-Pugh class C and varices, higher bilirubin levels, and lower serum sodium in this study, which might justify these differences.

Furthermore, nearly half of the patients were treated with a high-dose propranolol of 160 mg reported by Serste et al. However, a real-world multicenter study found that low-dose (≤80 mg/d) NSBBs treatment was associated with improved survival in primary and secondary prophylaxis of VB among advanced cirrhosis [37]. Park et al. also showed that low-dose propranolol (40–120 mg/d) decreased the risk of rebleeding of varices and mortality in patients with refractory ascites [38].

The window hypothesis, as proposed by Krag et al., suggests that the benefit windows of NSBBs may be closed once patients develop refractory ascites [17]. It may be explained that proinflammatory cytokines are increased in the splanchnic compartment among patients with refractory ascites, in whom chronic inflammation may cause decreased expression of β-adrenergic receptors and sympathetic nerve fiber loss, thereby leading to diminished effects of NSBBs [39]. However, several recent studies to investigate the efficacy of NSBBs in patients with ascites have reported opposite results. Tergast et al. enrolled 624 decompensated cirrhotic patients with ascites to evaluate the impact of NSBBs on survival. It showed that the administration of NSBBs is associated with improved 28-day transplant-free survival [40]. Leithead et al. included 322 patients with ascites who were listed for liver transplantation and identified significantly lower waiting-list mortality in NSBBs group [41]. Additionally, Onali et al. and Facciorusso et al. did not demonstrate that NSBBs affected the overall survival in cirrhotic patients with refractory ascites [42, 43].

Notably, the guideline for the management of ascites in cirrhosis by the British Society of Gastroenterology suggests that refractory ascites should not be considered a contraindication of NSBBs [44]. Patients with refractory ascites who are taking NSBBs should be closely monitored, and if they develop hypotension or acute/progressive renal dysfunction, the dosage may be reduced or discontinued appropriately. Similarly, the Baveno VII consensus proposed that NSBBs should be discontinued or decreased in patients with ascites who develop sustained hypotension (systolic blood pressure < 90 mmHg or mean arterial blood pressure < 65 mmHg) and/or hepato-renal syndrome-acute kidney injury (HRS-AKI). Once blood pressure returns to baseline and/or HRS-AKI resolves, NSBBs should be restarted [12]. In conclusion, the current evidence would not support discontinuation of NSBBs in patients with ascites or refractory ascites. NSBBs should be used with careful attention and reduced or discontinued in those, if appropriate.

3.3 NSBBs and renal dysfunction

Serste et al. included 139 patients with severe hepatitis to estimate the effect of NSBBs on the risk of development of AKI, in which the cumulative AKI incidence was significantly higher in the NSBBs group than in the non-NSBBs group (89.6 vs. 50.4%, P = 0.0001). They concluded that NSBBs were an independent risk factor for AKI in those patients [45]. Kim et al. identified that the impact of NSBBs on renal injury varied according to the severity of hepatic decompensation, with an increased risk of AKI by more than three-fold in cirrhotic patients with ascites [46]. Meanwhile, Singh et al. evaluated the effect of NSBBs on the development of AKI and 12-month transplant-free-survival in patients with ≥grade 2 ascites compared to EVL. They observed that the use of NSBBs is associated with poor survival and increased risk of AKI in those patients [47]. Finally, a meta-analysis including 14 studies, as reported by Xu et al., found that NSBBs significantly increased the risk of developing renal dysfunction [48]. The explanation for this apparent discrepancy lies in the fact that renal perfusion and its function are dependent on excessive activation of the sympathetic nervous system in patients with advanced cirrhosis, while NSBBs blunt the sympathetic overdrive, reduce cardiac output, and decrease renal perfusion pressures below critical values, thereby impairing renal function [49]. Notably, Xu et al. failed to demonstrate the association of NSBBs with an increased risk of development of renal dysfunction after covariate adjustment. Bang et al. and Scheiner et al. also found that treatment with NSBBs was associated neither with impairing of kidney function nor with increased incidence of AKI [50, 51].

However, Li et al. showed that the administration of NSBBs may reduce the occurrence of AKI and marginally alleviate chronic renal function declination [52]. Maiwall et al. observed consecutive cirrhotic patients with a complete record of baseline hemodynamics. During a median follow-up of 379 days, they found that treatment with NSBBs could prevent the frequency of AKI and the development of chronic kidney disease (CKD) [53]. It may be attributed to the fact that PH and severe vasodilation predispose cirrhotic patients to repeatedly develop AKI and progression to CKD, while NSBBs could improve hemodynamic response and reduce portal pressure, thereby decreasing the occurrence of AKI and CKD. Thus, the current evidence regarding the impact of NSBBs on renal dysfunction remains controversial. According to updated guidelines and consensus, NSBBs should be discontinued or dose-reduced in patients who develop AKI and CKD [12, 13].

3.4 NSBBs and spontaneous bacterial peritonitis

A meta-analysis included six studies to evaluate the possible role of NSBBs in spontaneous bacterial peritonitis (SBP) among cirrhotic patients with ascites, which found that NSBBs reduced the risk of SBP in the whole cohort, and the effect is still observed when compared between hemodynamic responders and non-responders [54]. It may be attributed to the non-hemodynamic mechanisms of NSBBs in reducing bacterial translocation and inflammatory response [55]. A large-scale retrospective cohort study from Denmark included 361 patients with SBP and revealed that the use of NSBBs was associated with improved survival. Additionally, in patients with severe decompensated cirrhosis, the use of NSBBs was associated with a lower risk of occurrence of SBP [50]. A prospective cohort study evaluated the possible factors associated with the prediction of recurrent SBP, which found that nonuse of prophylactic NSBBs was strongly associated with an increased rate of SBP recurrence [56].

However, Mandorfer et al. showed that treatment with NSBBs may be associated with poor transplant-free survival, increased risk of HRS and AKI, and extended periods of hospitalization in patients with SBP [57]. Notably, the NSBBs group had a higher bilirubin level, and a higher proportion of Child-Pugh class C and varices among SBP patients for subgroup analysis in this study might justify these differences. Similarly, according to the European Association for the Study of the Liver (EASL) clinical practice guideline, NSBBs should be discontinued in patients with acute complications such as VB, sepsis, SBP, or AKI. After recovery, it may be reinitiated appropriately [13]. Currently, controversy remains regarding the definitive efficacy of NSBBs in patients with SBP, but it is recommended to discontinue the use of NSBBs once the patients develop SBP. In future, large-scale prospective studies are needed to further explore the relationship between NSBBs and SBP.

3.5 NSBBs and portal vein thrombosis

Portal vein thrombosis (PVT) is mainly associated with decreased portal vein blood flow and velocity, and the portal vein blood flow <15 cm/s is considered an independent risk factor of PVT [58, 59]. The development of PVT is strongly associated with poor prognosis in cirrhotic patients [60, 61]. A significant higher risk of VB was observed in patients with PVT due to further increased portal pressure (47.33 vs. 19.63%) [62]. Currently, NSBBs are the first-line treatment for the prevention of VB, which significantly decrease the portal blood velocity and portal vein pressure [12]. However, Xu et al. indicated that a higher incidence of PVT was observed in the NSBBs group compared to the non-NSBBs group in univariate logistic regression analyses (P = 0.035), but no significant difference was found between the two groups after covariate adjustment (P = 0.194) [63]. Pan et al. demonstrated that decreased portal flow velocity and use of NSBBs were associated with the occurrence of PVT in liver cirrhosis [64]. Meanwhile, a meta-analysis included nine studies to evaluate whether NSBBs increase the risk of PVT, which found that the use of NSBBs increased a 4.62-fold risk of PVT in cirrhotic patients, but the results are limited by poor quality of included studies and significant heterogeneity across studies [65]. Therefore, there is inconclusive evidence to support the association of PVT formation with NSBBs, which requires large-scale RCTs to further confirm in the future.

4. Conclusion

NSBBs are the cornerstone for the management of PH in clinical practice, which has been specifically recommended for the primary and secondary prophylaxis of VB. In addition, the patient should be initiated on NSBBs promptly after the diagnosis of CSPH, regardless of the status of the varices. Considering the hemodynamic response of patients to NSBBs in cirrhosis varies based on the spectrum of cirrhosis, physicians should comprehensively assess the disease conditions of patients in clinical practice to choose the appropriate time and duration of administration with NSBBs.

Additionally, patients with ascites and refractory ascites should not be considered to be contraindications for NSBBs, which should be used under careful monitoring. Notably, if patients persistently develop hypotension and/or HRS-AKI, NSBBs should be discontinued or decreased until their blood pressure returns or HRS-AKI resolves, then restarted.

Author details

Ting Wang[1,2†], Cai'e Wang[1,2†], Hongyu Li[1,2*] and Ran Wang[1*]

1 Department of Gastroenterology, General Hospital of Northern Theater Command (Teaching Hospital of Shenyang Pharmaceutical University), Shenyang, China

2 Postgraduate College, Shenyang Pharmaceutical University, Shenyang, China

*Address all correspondence to: 13309887041@163.com and wangran891017@163.com

† Contributed equally to this work.

References

[1] Premkumar M, Anand AC. Overview of complications in cirrhosis. Journal of Clinical and Experimental Hepatology. 2022;**12**(4):1150-1174

[2] Iwakiri Y, Trebicka J. Portal hypertension in cirrhosis: Pathophysiological mechanisms and therapy. JHEP Reports: Innovation in Hepatology. 2021;**3**(4):100316

[3] Mauro E, Gadano A. What's new in portal hypertension? Liver International: Official Journal of the International Association for the Study of the Liver. 2020;**40**(Suppl 1):122-127

[4] Sauerbruch T, Schierwagen R, Trebicka J. Managing portal hypertension in patients with liver cirrhosis. F1000Research. 2 May 2018;7:F1000 Faculty Rev-533

[5] Guixé-Muntet S, Quesada-Vázquez S, Gracia-Sancho J. Pathophysiology and therapeutic options for cirrhotic portal hypertension. The Lancet Gastroenterology & Hepatology. 17 Apr 2024:S2468-1253(23)00438-7

[6] Shukla A, Kale A. Hyperdynamic circulation in cirrhosis: A novel gutsy central neuronal mechanism. Hepatology International. 2023;**17**(3):517-518

[7] Rodrigues SG, Mendoza YP, Bosch J. Beta-blockers in cirrhosis: Evidence-based indications and limitations. JHEP Reports: Innovation in Hepatology. 2020;**2**(1):100063

[8] McDonald N, Lilburn DML, Lachlan NJ, et al. Assessment of haemodynamic response to nonselective beta-blockers in portal hypertension by phase-contrast magnetic resonance angiography. BioMed Research International. 2017;**2017**:9281450

[9] Bosch J, Iwakiri Y. The portal hypertension syndrome: Etiology, classification, relevance, and animal models. Hepatology International. 2018;**12**(Suppl. 1):1-10

[10] Tittanegro T, China L, Forrest E, et al. Use of non-selective B-blockers is safe in hospitalised decompensated cirrhosis patients and exerts a potential anti-inflammatory effect: Data from the ATTIRE trial. EClinicalMedicine. 2023;**55**:101716

[11] Kockerling D, Nathwani R, Forlano R, Manousou P, Mullish BH, Dhar A. Current and future pharmacological therapies for managing cirrhosis and its complications. World Journal of Gastroenterology. 2019;**25**(8):888-908

[12] De Franchis R, Bosch J, Garcia-Tsao G, Reiberger T, Ripoll C, Baveno VIIF. Baveno VII—Renewing consensus in portal hypertension. Journal of Hepatology. 2022;**76**(4):959-974

[13] European Association for the Study of the Liver. EASL Clinical Practice Guidelines for the management of patients with decompensated cirrhosis. Journal of Hepatology. Aug 2018;**69**(2):406-460

[14] Yoshiji H, Nagoshi S, Akahane T, et al. Evidence-based clinical practice guidelines for liver cirrhosis 2020. Hepatology Research. 2021;**51**(7):725-749

[15] Cales P, Bertrais S, Boursier J, Fouchard I, Oberti F, Group S. Non-selective beta-blockers increase overall and liver mortality in alcoholic

cirrhosis with MELD >/= 12 over 5 years of follow-up. Liver International: Official Journal of the International Association for the Study of the Liver. 2021;**41**(1):168-179

[16] Tonon M, D'Ambrosio R, Calvino V, et al. A new clinical and prognostic characterization of the patterns of decompensation of cirrhosis. Journal of Hepatology. 2024;**80**(4):603-609

[17] Krag A, Wiest R, Albillos A, Gluud LL. The window hypothesis: Haemodynamic and non-haemodynamic effects of beta-blockers improve survival of patients with cirrhosis during a window in the disease. Gut. 2012;**61**(7):967-969

[18] Vorobioff JD, Groszmann RJ. Prevention of portal hypertension: From variceal development to clinical decompensation. Hepatology (Baltimore, Md). 2015;**61**(1):375-381

[19] Zanetto A, Barbiero G, Battistel M, et al. Management of portal hypertension severe complications. Minerva Gastroenterol (Torino). 2021;**67**(1):26-37

[20] Villanueva C, Albillos A, Genescà J, et al. β blockers to prevent decompensation of cirrhosis in patients with clinically significant portal hypertension (PREDESCI): A randomised, double-blind, placebo-controlled, multicentre trial. Lancet (London, England). 2019;**393**(10181):1597-1608

[21] Villanueva C, Torres F, Sarin SK, et al. Carvedilol reduces the risk of decompensation and mortality in patients with compensated cirrhosis in a competing-risk meta-analysis. Journal of Hepatology. 2022;**77**(4):1014-1025

[22] Kumar M, Kainth S, Choudhury A, et al. Treatment with carvedilol improves survival of patients with acute-on-chronic liver failure: A randomized controlled trial. Hepatology International. 2019;**13**(6):800-813

[23] Reiberger T, Ulbrich G, Ferlitsch A, et al. Carvedilol for primary prophylaxis of variceal bleeding in cirrhotic patients with haemodynamic non-response to propranolol. Gut. 2013;**62**(11):1634-1641

[24] McDowell HR, Chuah CS, Tripathi D, Stanley AJ, Forrest EH, Hayes PC. Carvedilol is associated with improved survival in patients with cirrhosis: A long-term follow-up study. Alimentary Pharmacology & Therapeutics. 2021;**53**(4):531-539

[25] Sharma M, Singh S, Desai V, et al. Comparison of therapies for primary prevention of esophageal variceal bleeding: A systematic review and network meta-analysis. Hepatology (Baltimore, Md). 2019;**69**(4):1657-1675

[26] Villanueva C, Albillos A, Genesca J, et al. Development of hyperdynamic circulation and response to beta-blockers in compensated cirrhosis with portal hypertension. Hepatology (Baltimore, Md). 2016;**63**(1):197-206

[27] Bultas AC, Teshome B, Richter SK, Schafers S, Cooke E, Call WB. Use of nonselective β-blockers in patients with end-stage liver disease and select complications. The Annals of Pharmacotherapy. 2020;**54**(6):583-593

[28] Villanueva C, Sapena V, Lo GH, et al. Improving primary prophylaxis of variceal bleeding by adapting therapy to the clinical stage of cirrhosis. A competing-risk meta-analysis of individual participant data. Alimentary Pharmacology & Therapeutics. 2024;**59**(3):306-321

[29] Kong Y, Shi L. Comparison of the effectiveness of 11 mainstay

treatments for secondary prophylaxis of variceal bleeding in patients with cirrhosis: A network meta-analysis. Experimental and Therapeutic Medicine. 2020;**19**(6):3479-3496

[30] Shi L, Zhang X, Li J, Bai X. Favorable effects of endoscopic ligation combined with drugs on rebleeding and mortality in cirrhotic patients: A network meta-analysis. Digestive Diseases. 2018;**36**(2):136-149

[31] Jachs M, Hartl L, Simbrunner B, et al. Carvedilol achieves higher hemodynamic response and lower rebleeding rates than propranolol in secondary prophylaxis. Clinical Gastroenterology and Hepatology: The Official Clinical Practice Journal of the American Gastroenterological Association. 2022

[32] Groszmann RJ, Garcia-Tsao G, Bosch J, et al. Beta-blockers to prevent gastroesophageal varices in patients with cirrhosis. The New England Journal of Medicine. 2005;**353**(21):2254-2261

[33] Qi XS, Bao YX, Bai M, Xu WD, Dai JN, Guo XZ. Nonselective beta-blockers in cirrhotic patients with no or small varices: A meta-analysis. World Journal of Gastroenterology. 2015;**21**(10):3100-3108

[34] Bhardwaj A, Kedarisetty CK, Vashishtha C, et al. Carvedilol delays the progression of small oesophageal varices in patients with cirrhosis: A randomised placebo-controlled trial. Gut. 2017;**66**(10):1838-1843

[35] Di Pascoli L, Buja A, Bolognesi M, et al. Cost-effectiveness analysis of beta-blockers vs endoscopic surveillance in patients with cirrhosis and small varices. World Journal of Gastroenterology. 2014;**20**(30):10464-10469

[36] Serste T, Melot C, Francoz C, et al. Deleterious effects of beta-blockers on survival in patients with cirrhosis and refractory ascites. Hepatology (Baltimore, Md). 2010;**52**(3):1017-1022

[37] Kang SH, Lee M, Kim MY, et al. The longitudinal outcomes of applying non-selective beta-blockers in portal hypertension: Real-world multicenter study. Hepatology International. 2021;**15**(2):424-436

[38] Park JH, Jun DW, Choi J, et al. Low-dose propranolol as secondary prophylaxis for varix bleeding decreases mortality and rebleeding rate in patients with tense ascites. Journal of Clinical Medicine. 2019;**8**(5)

[39] Almenara S, Lozano B, Gimenez P, et al. Functionality of beta-adrenergic receptors in patients with cirrhosis treated chronically with non-selective beta-blockers. Hepatology International. 2020;**14**(5):858-868

[40] Tergast TL, Kimmann M, Laser H, et al. Systemic arterial blood pressure determines the therapeutic window of non-selective beta blockers in decompensated cirrhosis. Alimentary Pharmacology & Therapeutics. 2019;**50**(6):696-706

[41] Leithead JA, Rajoriya N, Tehami N, et al. Non-selective β-blockers are associated with improved survival in patients with ascites listed for liver transplantation. Gut. 2015;**64**(7):1111-1119

[42] Onali S, Kalafateli M, Majumdar A, et al. Non-selective beta-blockers are not associated with increased mortality in cirrhotic patients with ascites. Liver International: Official Journal of the International Association for the Study of the Liver. 2017;**37**(9):1334-1344

[43] Facciorusso A, Roy S, Livadas S, et al. Nonselective beta-blockers do not affect survival in cirrhotic patients with

ascites. Digestive Diseases and Sciences. 2018;**63**(7):1737-1746

[44] Aithal GP, Palaniyappan N, China L, et al. Guidelines on the management of ascites in cirrhosis. Gut. 2021;**70**(1):9-29

[45] Serste T, Njimi H, Degre D, et al. The use of beta-blockers is associated with the occurrence of acute kidney injury in severe alcoholic hepatitis. Liver International: Official Journal of the International Association for the Study of the Liver. 2015;**35**(8):1974-1982

[46] Kim SG, Larson JJ, Lee JS, Therneau TM, Kim WR. Beneficial and harmful effects of nonselective beta blockade on acute kidney injury in liver transplant candidates. Liver Transplantation. 2017;**23**(6):733-740

[47] Singh V, Kumar P, Verma N, Vijayvergiya R, Singh A, Bhalla A. Propranolol vs. band ligation for primary prophylaxis of variceal hemorrhage in cirrhotic patients with ascites: A randomized controlled trial. Hepatology International. 2022;**16**(4):944-953

[48] Xu X, Gao F, Wang T, Yang Z, Zhao Q, Qi X. Association of non-selective beta blockers with the development of renal dysfunction in liver cirrhosis: A systematic review and meta-analysis. Annals of Medicine. 2024;**56**(1):2305935

[49] Tellez L, Albillos A. Non-selective beta-blockers in patients with ascites: The complex interplay among the liver, kidney and heart. Liver International: Official Journal of the International Association for the Study of the Liver. 2022;**42**(4):749-761

[50] Bang UC, Benfield T, Hyldstrup L, Jensen JE, Bendtsen F. Effect of propranolol on survival in patients with decompensated cirrhosis: A nationwide study based Danish patient registers. Liver International: Official Journal of the International Association for the Study of the Liver. 2016;**36**(9):1304-1312

[51] Scheiner B, Parada-Rodriguez D, Bucsics T, et al. Non-selective beta-blocker treatment does not impact on kidney function in cirrhotic patients with varices. Scandinavian Journal of Gastroenterology. 2017;**52**(9):1008-1015

[52] Li TH, Liu CW, Huang CC, et al. Non-selective beta-blockers decrease infection, acute kidney injury episodes, and ameliorate sarcopenic changes in patients with cirrhosis: A propensity-score matching tertiary-center cohort study. Journal of Clinical Medicine. 2021;**10**(11)

[53] Maiwall R, Pasupuleti SSR, Jain P, Sarin SK. Degree of portal and systemic hemodynamic alterations predict recurrent AKI and chronic kidney disease in patients with cirrhosis. Hepatology Communications. 2021;**5**(2):293-308

[54] Senzolo M, Cholongitas E, Burra P, et al. Beta-blockers protect against spontaneous bacterial peritonitis in cirrhotic patients: A meta-analysis. Liver International: Official Journal of the International Association for the Study of the Liver. 2009;**29**(8):1189-1193

[55] Mookerjee RP, Pavesi M, Thomsen KL, et al. Treatment with non-selective beta blockers is associated with reduced severity of systemic inflammation and improved survival of patients with acute-on-chronic liver failure. Journal of Hepatology. 2016;**64**(3):574-582

[56] Abdel-Razik A, Abdelsalam M, Gad DF, Abdelwahab A, Tawfik M, Elzehery R, et al. Recurrence of spontaneous bacterial peritonitis in cirrhosis: Novel predictors. European

Journal of Gastroenterology & Hepatology. Jun 2020;**32**(6):718-726

[57] Mandorfer M, Bota S, Schwabl P, et al. Nonselective beta blockers increase risk for hepatorenal syndrome and death in patients with cirrhosis and spontaneous bacterial peritonitis. Gastroenterology. 2014;**146**(7):1680-1690 e1681

[58] Senzolo M, Garcia-Tsao G, Garcia-Pagan JC. Current knowledge and management of portal vein thrombosis in cirrhosis. Journal of Hepatology. 2021;**75**(2):442-453

[59] Harding DJ, Perera MT, Chen F, Olliff S, Tripathi D. Portal vein thrombosis in cirrhosis: Controversies and latest developments. World Journal of Gastroenterology. 2015;**21**(22):6769-6784

[60] Qi X, Bai M, Yang Z, et al. Occlusive portal vein thrombosis as a new marker of decompensated cirrhosis. Medical Hypotheses. 2011;**76**(4):522-526

[61] Zhang Y, Xu BY, Wang XB, et al. Prevalence and clinical significance of portal vein thrombosis in patients with cirrhosis and acute decompensation. Clinical Gastroenterology and Hepatology: The Official Clinical Practice Journal of the American Gastroenterological Association. 2020;**18**(11):2564-2572 e2561

[62] Qi X, Su C, Ren W, et al. Association between portal vein thrombosis and risk of bleeding in liver cirrhosis: A systematic review of the literature. Clinics and Research in Hepatology and Gastroenterology. 2015;**39**(6):683-691

[63] Xu X, Xu S, Primignani M, et al. Nonselective beta-blockers may progress the thrombosis of portal venous system in cirrhotic patients: A retrospective observational study. Advances in Therapy. 2020;**37**(4):1452-1463

[64] Pan J, Wang L, Gao F, et al. Epidemiology of portal vein thrombosis in liver cirrhosis: A systematic review and meta-analysis. European Journal of Internal Medicine. 2022;**104**:21-32

[65] Xu X, Guo X, De Stefano V, et al. Nonselective beta-blockers and development of portal vein thrombosis in liver cirrhosis: A systematic review and meta-analysis. Hepatology International. 2019;**13**(4):468-481

Chapter 4

Role of Transarterial Radioembolization in Management of HCC

Wali Badar, Ali Husnain, John Fung and Osman Ahmed

Abstract

Transarterial Radioembolization (TARE) is an emerging therapy for the management of hepatocellular carcinoma (HCC). Radioactive Y90 can be loaded onto glass or resin microparticles for intra-arterial selective internal radiation therapy. TARE is a multistage procedure requiring a mapping procedure and a treatment procedure. The mapping procedure informs operators on vascular anatomy as well as potential arteriovenous shunting. Based on the device desired, goal of treatment, vascularity of the tumor and shunting, dosage can be computed for treatment day. Overall, TARE is generally a well-tolerated procedure with promising clinical outcomes with HCC for the purposes of curative therapy, downstaging, and palliation.

Keywords: hepatocellular carcinoma (HCC), Yttrium 90 (Y90), TARE, locoregional therapy (LRT), dosimetry, interventional oncology (IO), Technetium 99m macro aggregated albumin (Tc-99m MAA) mapping, Therasphere®, SIR-Sphere®

1. Introduction

HCC the most common primary liver cancer and has the fourth highest cancer-related mortality [1, 2]. The five-year survival rate of primary liver cancer is second lowest to only pancreatic cancer [3]. For early-stage disease, surgical resection and orthotopic liver transplant represent curative options but a large majority of patients are poor surgical candidates or transplant ineligible. For unresectable early-stage disease, percutaneous ablation can achieve outcomes similar to surgical resection [4]. For intermediate-stage disease, transarterial chemoembolization (TACE) offers improved survival benefits. For advanced-stage disease, systemic therapy offers modest benefits.

Transarterial radioembolization (TARE) with Yttrium 90 (Y90) is a popular and relatively new locoregional therapy (LRT) for unresectable hepatocellular carcinoma (HCC). Strategies for use include curative intent, downstaging and/or bridging to liver transplantation, and palliation. As such, TARE has role for management in HCC for unresectable early, intermediate, and advanced-stage disease. This chapter reviews TARE treatment selection amongst various LRTs in addition to treatment planning, dosimetry, safety and efficacy data, and therapeutic applications.

2. HCC and the treatment paradigm

HCC is a major world health issue, with 750,000 new cases a year and the incidence is expected to continue to rise with the rise of hepatitis C and obesity/non-alcoholic hepatic steatosis [1]. The Barcelona Clinic Liver Cancer (BCLC) system is a widely accepted staging system for HCC management, seen in **Figure 1**. The 2022 Update of the BCLC treatment algorithm offered an expanded role for TARE [4]. For early stage (A), TARE is used for unresectable disease in order to bridge patients for transplant. For intermediate stage disease (B), transarterial therapies including TACE and TARE are used. TARE has demonstrated longer time to progression compared to TACE (>26 months vs 6.8 months, $p = 0.0012$) in a randomized phase 2 study (PREMIERE) [5]. Furthermore, TARE has demonstrated a favorable adverse event profile, lower incidence of diarrhea (0% vs 21%, $p = 0.031$) and hypoalbuminemia (4% vs 58%, $p < 0.001$), and increased quality of life compared to TACE using subjective measures of social well-being, functional well-being, and embolotherapy specific toxicities [5, 6]. Lastly for advanced stage (C), TARE has shown comparable survival benefits compared to Sorafenib, a systemic chemotherapeutic, with respect to overall survival (8.0 vs 9.9 months, $p = 0.18$) and improved treatment tolerance with twice as many adverse events with Sorafenib in the SARAH randomized control trial [7]. The focus of the next section will be an overview of the pathophysiology and different devices used with TARE.

2.1 Pathophysiology of TARE and current devices

Transarterial radioembolization (TARE) is a form of selective internal radiation therapy described as transcatheter intra-arterial delivery of radioactive microparticles for the treatment of primary or secondary liver cancer [8]. While normal hepatic parenchyma derives >70% of its blood supply from the portal vein, primary HCC receives greater than 90% of its tumoral blood supply from the hepatic artery by way of neo-angiogenesis. This principle is utilized in TARE to safely deliver radioactive

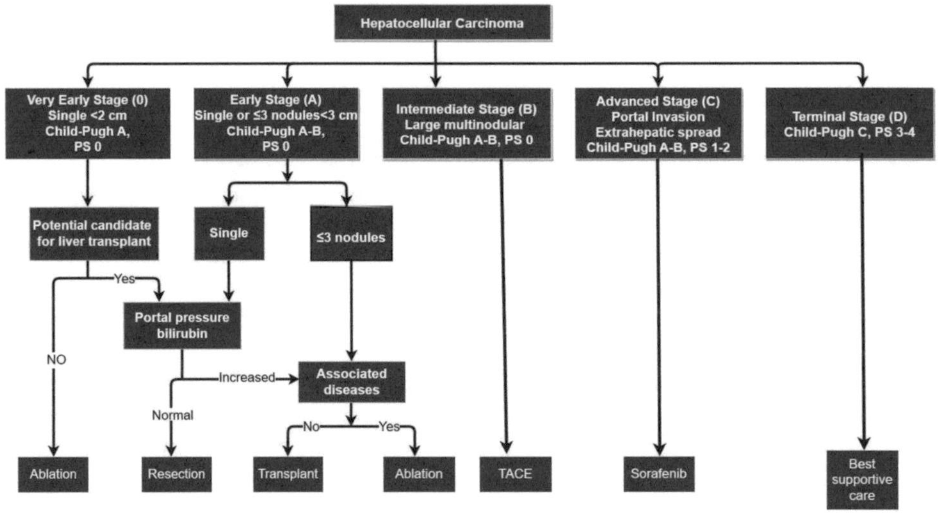

Figure 1.
BCLC staging system for treatment of HCC.

Glass microspheres	Resin microspheres
Diameter of 20–30 μm and activity of 2500 Bq per sphere [8].	Diameter of 20–60 μm and activity of 50 Bq per sphere [9].
1.2 million glass microspheres produce an activity of 3 GBq (2500 Bq per sphere) [8].	40–80 million resin microspheres produce an activity of 3 GBq (50 Bq per sphere) [8].
Indications: • Unresectable HCC • HCC complicated by PVT [12].	**Indications:** • Unresectable colorectal metastases in combination with chemotherapy (fludarabine) [8].
Given the greater specific activity of Y90 per microsphere, the desired dose delivery is possible without embolizing the blood vessel [13].	Due to the lower specific activity of each microsphere, it is difficult to deliver the desired dose without embolizing the blood vessel [14].

Table 1.
Summary of Y90 devices which include glass and resin microspheres.

microparticles to the tumor without affecting the surrounding liver [9]. Since the PREMIERE trial in 2016, there has been further investigation and increased acceptance of TARE as a key treatment modality for HCC [5]. Yttrium-90 (Y90) is the radioactive isotope most often used in TARE. Y90 has a half-life of 64.2 h and emits pure β particles (cytotoxic to tumor cells) as it decays into Zirconium-90. The average tissue penetration of Y90 is 2.5 mm with a maximum of 11 mm. This narrow range of penetrance is important for local tissue delivery with sparing of the surrounding liver tissue [10, 11]. There are two main devices for loading of the radioactive isotope to microparticles: resin and glass microspheres which are commercially produced by SIR-spheres® (Sirtex Medical, Woburn, MA, USA) and TheraSphere® (Boston Scientific, Marlborough, MA, USA), respectively [8]. Glass microspheres are US Food and Drug Administration (FDA)-approved for the treatment of unresectable HCC or HCC complicated by portal vein invasion [12]. The porous nature of glass microspheres allows for higher loading dose of Y90 per sphere making it a suitable candidate for locally delivering the desired radiation dose without a detectable embolizing effect [8, 13]. On the other hand, resin microspheres have lower radiation dose per sphere as the radioisotope is coated on the periphery of the sphere. Therefore, a higher quantity of spheres is required to deliver a desired dose, increasing risk for stasis of blood flow and embolization of the artery before completion of instillation [9, 14]. The two devices are summarized in **Table 1**.

2.2 Treatment planning

TARE is a two-step therapy consisting of a treatment-planning procedure ("mapping") followed by a separate intervention for Y90 administration. The mapping procedure is performed to identify the arterial supply of the treated tumor(s), assess for potential enterohepatic collaterals that may result in non-target embolization, as well as administering Technetium 99m macro aggregated albumin (Tc-99m MAA) to calculate the hepatopulmonary shunt fraction. The first stage entails hepatic angiography to evaluate the arterial anatomy. Roughly 45% of patients can have variant hepatic artery anatomy which can lead to nontarget delivery of Y90 to tissues such as the stomach, gallbladder, and bowel if not properly accounted for [15]. The common hepatic artery usually arises at the celiac trifurcation along with the left gastric artery and splenic artery. After the takeoff of the gastroduodenal artery, the common hepatic

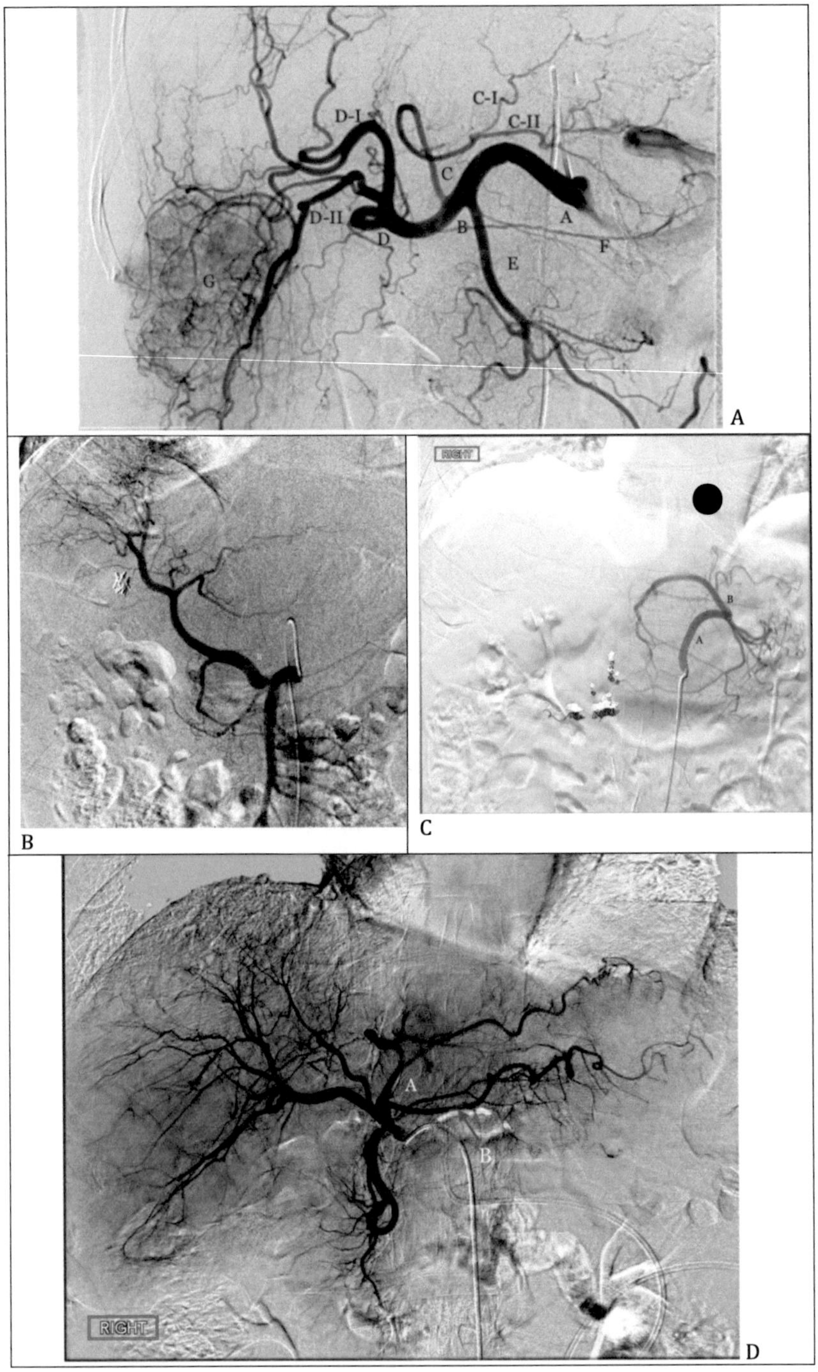

Figure 2.
A: Digital subtraction angiogram (DSA) of the common hepatic artery (A) with branches labeled as followed: B = proper hepatic artery; C = left hepatic artery (C-I = lat. branch of left hepatic artery; C-II = med. branch of left hepatic artery); D = right hepatic artery (D-I = ant. branch of right hepatic artery; D-II = post. branch of right hepatic artery); E = gastroduodenal artery; F = right gastric artery; G = Arterially enhancing tumor; B: DSA of replaced right hepatic artery (A) arising off of superior mesenteric artery (B); C: DSA of replaced left hepatic artery (B) arising off of the left gastric artery (A); D: DSA of accessory left gastric artery arising off of the left hepatic artery.

artery gives rise to the proper haptic artery which bifurcates into the right and left hepatic arteries. The two most common variations of the hepatic arterial vasculature include the replaced right hepatic artery arising from the superior mesenteric artery and the replaced left hepatic artery arising from the left gastric artery (**Figure 2**) [15]. Next, it is important to evaluate the origin of vessels such as the right gastric artery which typically arises from the proper hepatic artery but can arise off the left hepatic artery. If radioactive microparticles are administered proximal to the takeoff of the right gastric artery, severe radiation-induced gastric ulcerations can result [16]. Other vessels that can result in nontarget delivery of Y90 include the gastroduodenal, cystic, falciform, left inferior phrenic, and supraduodenal arteries [17]. Additionally, accessory arteries such as the accessory left gastric artery can arise from the left hepatic artery and cause nontarget embolization (**Figure 2**).

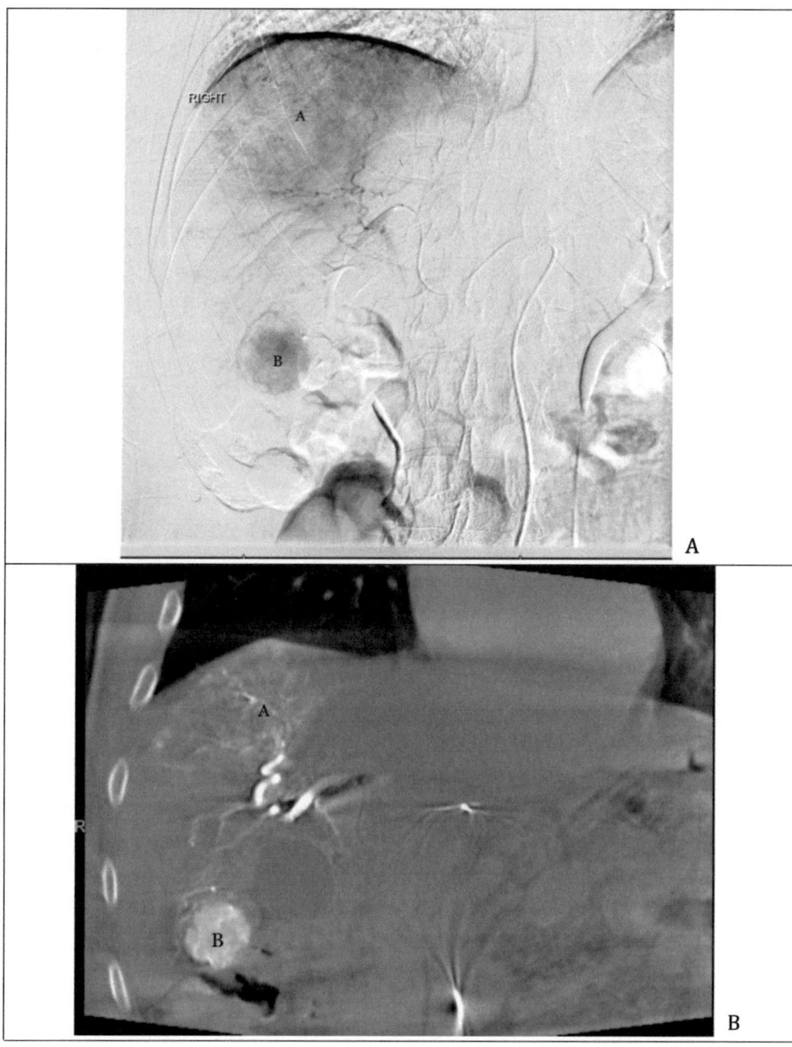

Figure 3.
A: DSA demonstrating arterially enhancing tumors; B: Cone Beam CT correlate from DSA assuring tumor has adequete arterial coverage.

Nontarget vessels can be coiled off during the mapping procedure if the catheter cannot be positioned beyond the vessel origin for treatment. In addition to evaluating for causes of nontarget embolization, angiography is used to identify which arteries need to be treated to provide adequate arterial coverage. Typically, intra-procedure cross sectional imaging such as cone beam CT is performed to confirm arterial coverage as seen in **Figure 3**.

Once arterial coverage is confirmed, Tc-99m MAA is delivered via microcatheter at the expected site of treatment. Tc-99m MAA is used to predict the distribution of Y90 on treatment day as it has similar tissue penetrance as Y90 with significantly lower activity [18]. After infusion of Tc-99m MAA, detection of gamma radiation is used to evaluate radioactive microparticle distribution with Single Photon Emission Computed Tomography (SPECT). The planar imaging (with or without accompanying CT) is compared to mapping angiography to assess if the bulk of gamma radiation counts are localized to area of local injection. At this time, nontarget delivery of MAA can be assessed by evaluation radioactivity in the stomach and bowel. In addition to accessory vasculature leading to nontarget embolization, reflux of microparticles during MAA can also contribute to extrahepatic delivery. Planar imaging can also be used to compute the hepatopulmonary ("lung shunt") fraction by calculating the arithmetic or geometric mean of radioactivity counts with in the lung, using anterior and posterior projections, compared to the sum of counts in the liver and the lungs. Arteriovenous shunts can provide a direct pathway for radioactive microparticles to traverse from the liver to the lung leading to radiation pneumonitis. Sample planar imaging is seen in **Figure 4** and the equation for assessing the lung shunt fraction is seen in equation 1. For glass microparticles there is a high association of radiation pneumonitis with doses of greater than 30 Gy per treatment or greater than 50 Gy cumulatively across all lifetime treatments [11]. For resin microparticles, a lung shunt fraction of less than 20% is recommended [11].

$$\text{LSF} = \frac{\text{Mean Lung Counts}}{\text{Mean Lung Counts} + \text{Mean Liver Counts}} \tag{1}$$

Equation 1. Equation for calculation of lung shunt fraction.

2.3 Dosimetry of TARE

Dosimetry refers to the dose determination process for TARE and takes into account many factors such as intent of therapy (i.e. curative vs palliative), tumor burden (segmental vs lobar), arteriovenous shunting/lung shunting, and patient size. Lobar or radiation lobectomy refers to treatment of 3 or more liver segments whereas "segmentectomy" refers to two or fewer segments as identified by the Couinad liver segmentation classification system [11]. Additionally, it is important to understand the difference between dosage as well as activity. Dosage refers to the amount of energy (Joules) imparted on a specific mass of tissue (kg) and is measured in gray (Gy). Activity is defined by the amount of energy that is lost per unit time by an isotope due to radioactive decay and is measured by Becquerel (Bq).

There are two main mathematic models that are used to calculate dosage which include the Medical Internal Radiation Dose (MIRD) model and the Partition model. Each of these models are summarized in Eq. (2) [11]. The MIRD is a single compartment model that assumes there is uniform distribution of activity into the desired tissue and the inputs are the desired dosage for treatment, mass of the liver, and the lung shunt fraction [11]. Historically, for lobar treatment with glass microspheres a

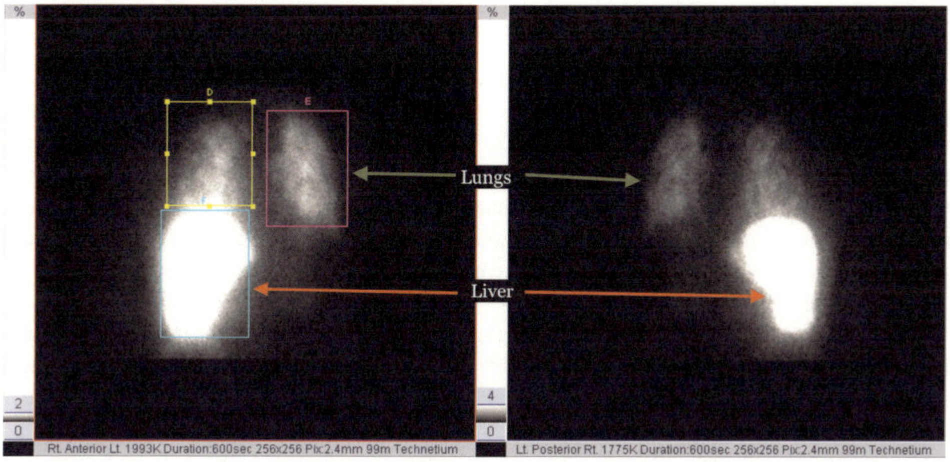

Figure 4.
Sample planar SPECT images showing radiation counts in the lungs and liver.

dosage of 120–150 Gy is used whereas segmental treatment dosing is done with target dosing >400 Gy using MIRD.

The Partition model assumes that the radioactive microparticles distribute into non-tumorous liver tissue as well as the intended tumor. The inputs of the Partition model include: the maximum dose that is desired to the healthy liver, the ratio of MAA uptake in the tumor vs the healthy liver which is determined by SPECT or SPECT CT, mass of tumor and normal liver tissue, and lastly the lung shunt fraction. MIRD model is used primarily for glass microparticles while the Partition model can be used for both microsphere types [19].

$$\text{A}: D_{liver}\,[Gy] = 50\left[\frac{J}{Gbq}\right] \times \frac{A_{total}[GBq]}{m_{liver}};\, D_{lung}[Gy] = 50\left[\frac{J}{Gbq}\right] \times \frac{A_{total}[Gbq]}{m_{lung}[kg]} \times LSF$$

$$B: D_{liver}[Gy] = \frac{50\left[\frac{J}{GBq}\right] \times (A_{total})[GBq] \times (1 - LSF)}{m_{non-tumor}[kg] + \frac{T}{N} \times (m_{tumor})[kg]} \quad (2)$$

Equation 2; A represents the MIRD model and B represents the partition model. A is activity, D is dose, m is mass, and LSF is lung shunt fraction.

Both of the above-mentioned equations can be used to compute total activity of Y90 needed for the intended dosage of therapy. When the microparticles are ordered, they are calibrated by activity and are usually in 3 GBq per vials for resin microparticles and 3, 5, 7, 10, 15, and 20 GBq vials for glass microparticles [11]. Each respective manufacturer reports a shelf life of 12 days for glass microparticles and 3 days for resin microparticles. Each particle, within the vial, has a specific activity which determines the overall vial activity. Each particle can either have a high specific activity or low specific activity. If a large tumor is being treated, more microparticles are needed and therefore lower specific activity microparticles are desired [19]. The opposite is true for smaller tumors where fewer microparticles with higher specific activity is optimal. Vials are selected based on patient specific dosage and tumor size as well as the exact date and time of treatment because of the radioactive decay of Y90. Resin microspheres are calibrated on treatment day while glass microspheres are calibrated in advance and must be administered at a specific time [20].

2.4 Treatment day

Patients typically return 1–2 weeks following the mapping procedure for Y90 administration. The microcatheter is placed into the tumor-feeding arteries that were identified on the mapping procedure. After Y90 administration, the catheters used for infusion as well as the administration apparatus are collected for radiation survey and disposed based on institutional radiation safety protocol [11]. Of note, there are no extra precautions advised to the patient and family members after TARE regarding external radiation exposure as Y90 is a pure beta emitter and the radiation is confined to the abdomen [21].

After the procedure, it is prudent to evaluate the radioactive microparticle distribution within the hepatic and extra-hepatic tissue, similar to the mapping procedure with Tc-99m MAA. SPECT-CT in addition Positron Emission Tomography (PET) can be used to visualized the radioisotope distribution. Y90 undergoes beta negative decay which produces bremsstrahlung photons that are detected in SPECT-CT and PET-CT imaging. SPECT-CT is more commonly performed for biodistribution evaluation however PET-CT is believed to provide more precise and accurate detection [11]. An example of SPECT-CT showing biodistribution within the right hepatic lobe after lobar infusion is seen in **Figure 5**.

2.5 Safety and efficacy of TARE

TARE with Y-90 is a generally safe and effective. Immediately after the procedure, patients may experience post embolization syndrome (PES) which is comprised of an array of symptoms including abdominal pain or discomfort, nausea, vomiting, and fatigue. PES is usually self-limiting and treatment is supportive [22].

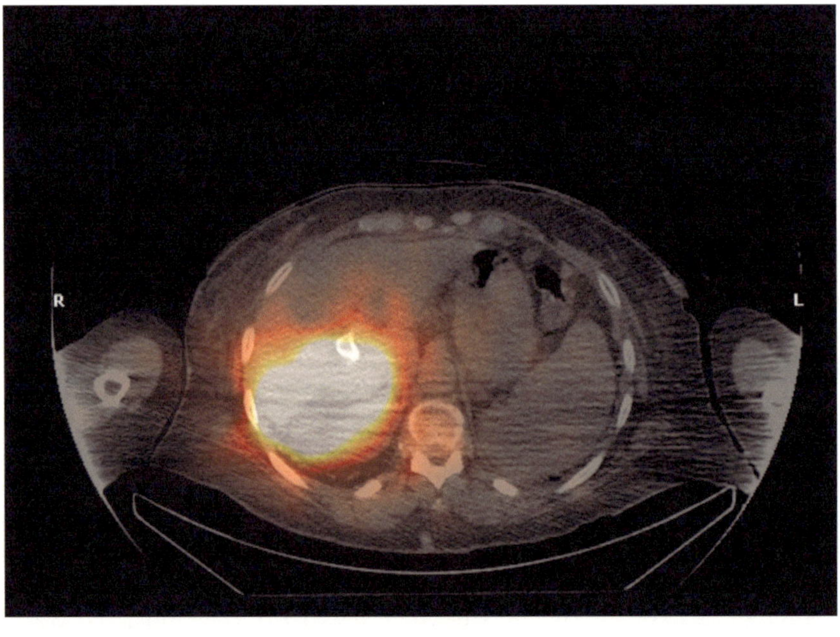

Figure 5.
Increased radiotracer uptake in the right hepatic lobe corresponding to treated region.

Radiation-induced liver disease (RILD) is one of the most feared adverse events related to TARE and occurs in less than 2% of the cases [23]. RILD is defined as new onset anicteric ascites with an increase in alkaline phosphatase that is out of proportion to other biliary enzymes within 2 months of TARE [24]. Repeat treatment with TARE has been demonstrated to be safe and effective in patients with residual or recurrent HCC [25].

Biliary complications are rare but include radiation cholecystitis, radiation-induced cholangitis, biliary necrosis, obstructive jaundice secondary to biliary strictures, and abscess/bilomas [23]. Pancreatic complications are uncommon and mostly include acute pancreatitis [23]. Pulmonary complications include radiation pneumonitis, atelectasis and pleural effusion. Gastrointestinal adverse events include diarrhea and mucosal ulceration which are consequences of nontarget embolization from hepatoenteric arterial communications [23].

The efficacy of TARE is assessed via cross-sectional abdominal imaging such as contrast-enhanced CT or MRI. Various imaging criteria exist to evaluate treatment response, including the modified Response Evaluation Criteria in Solid Tumors (mRECIST) and Liver Imaging Reporting and Data System (LI-RADS) [26, 27]. There is no set standard interval for post-TARE imaging, however, common practice is imaging at 1 month after the procedure, 3 months after the first follow-up scan, and then every 3–6 months afterwards [8].

2.6 Current applications of TARE

TARE has shown a multitude of benefits in various clinical scenarios which include curative therapy, bridging to transplant, and palliation. As mentioned earlier, the two main primary methods of TARE treatment include segmental or lobar treatments. Segmental infusions, described in literature as "radiation segmentectomy" is a growing area of clinical interest due to the ability for radiation dose escalation as Y90 microparticles are delivered to ≤2 segments of liver while sparing the rest of the liver. Lewandowski et al. first compared the outcomes of glass Y90 radiation segmentectomy, in patients with solitary tumors ≤5 cm, to other curative therapies such as surgical resection and radiofrequency ablation and found similar response rates, tumor control, and survival outcomes in tumors ≤3 cm, highlighting the curative potential of this approach [28]. Salem et al. investigated the utility of glass Y90 TARE for solitary tumors ≤ 8 cm in the multicenter LEGACY study [29]. The majority of patients received selective infusion and an 86.6% three-year overall survival rate was observed. Additionally, explanted livers showed complete pathological necrosis at doses greater than 400 Gy, establishing an ablative dose [29]. While TARE was initially thought to be an alternative to TACE in intermediate stage disease (BCLC stage B), the above-mentioned studies established the role of TARE in early-stage disease (BCLC stage 0 & A).

Lobar Y90 refers to treatment of an entire hepatic lobe via either the right or left hepatic artery. The dosage for lobectomy is usually lower than that of segmentectomy (120–150 Gy for glass microspheres), as there is a larger amount of radioactive microparticles delivered to the normal/non-tumorous surrounding liver parenchyma. A well-established phenomenon with high dose lobar Y90 is compensatory, contralateral hypertrophy of the remnant or untreated lobe [30]. This approach offers the advantage of local tumor control combined with a larger future liver remnant for those eligible for surgical resection. With the help of radiation lobectomy, the FLR (i.e. the untreated lobe) can increase by up to 45% of its original volume allowing for sufficient hepatic reserve to facilitate resection [31]. Lobar treatment has also shown benefit in advanced disease with portal vein tumor thrombus (PVTT) which is usually managed with systemic chemotherapy. Other LRTs including percutaneous ablation and TACE are not recommended for HCC with PVTT [7]. TACE is relatively contraindicated due to its embolic nature which could lead to hepatic infarction due to its embolic effect.

3. Conclusion

TARE is a safe and efficacious LRT that plays a large role in the treatment paradigm for HCC with applications in curative therapy, bridging to transplant, as well as palliation. TARE is a two-stage procedure that includes both a mapping procedure as well as the Y90 microparticle infusion. The mapping procedure informs operators on the vascular anatomy of the tumor as well as variant hepatic arterial anatomy, arteriovenous shunting, and hepatoenteric/hepatogastric collaterals. There are two general methods of TARE which include radiation segmentectomy and radiation lobectomy. Segmentectomy has outcomes similar to other curative procedures while lobectomy has shown utility in patients undergoing resection as well as in portal vein invasion.

Acknowledgements

We thank Omar Ahmad, Medical Student.

Conflict of interest

O.A. has received speaking fees from Argon Medical, Cook Medical, Cardiva Medical, and Canon Medical and has served on an advisory board for Boston Scientific and Genentech.

Author details

Wali Badar[1]*, Ali Husnain[2], John Fung[3] and Osman Ahmed[4]

1 Division of Interventional Radiology, Department of Radiology, University of Illinois Hospital and Health Sciences System, Chicago, IL, USA

2 Division of Interventional Radiology, Department of Radiology, Northwestern University, Chicago, IL, USA

3 Department of Surgery, Section of Transplant Surgery, University of Chicago, Chicago, IL, USA

4 Division of Interventional Radiology, Department of Radiology, University of Chicago, Chicago, IL, USA

*Address all correspondence to: wali94@gmail.com

References

[1] Villanueva A. Hepatocellular carcinoma. The New England Journal of Medicine. 2019;**380**(15):1450-1462. DOI: 10.1056/NEJMra1713263

[2] Philips CA, Rajesh S, Nair DC, Ahamed R, Abduljaleel JK, Augustine P. Hepatocellular carcinoma in 2021: An exhaustive update. Cureus. 2021;**13**(11): e19274. DOI: 10.7759/cureus.19274

[3] Rahib L, Wehner MR, Matrisian LM, Nead KT. Estimated projection of US cancer incidence and death to 2040. JAMA Network Open. 2021;**4**(4): e214708. DOI: 10.1001/jamanetworkopen.2021.4708

[4] Lucatelli P, Guiu B. 2022 update of BCLC treatment algorithm of HCC: What's new for interventional radiologists? Cardiovascular and Interventional Radiology. 2022;**45**(3): 275-276. DOI: 10.1007/s00270-021-03047-1

[5] Salem R, Gordon AC, Mouli S, Hickey R, Kallini J, Gabr A, et al. Y90 radioembolization significantly prolongs time to progression compared with chemoembolization in patients with hepatocellular carcinoma. Gastroenterology. 2016;**151**(6): 1155-1163.e2. DOI: 10.1053/j.gastro.2016.08.029

[6] Salem R, Gilbertsen M, Butt Z, Memon K, Vouche M, Hickey R, et al. Increased quality of life among hepatocellular carcinoma patients treated with radioembolization, compared with chemoembolization. Clinical Gastroenterology and Hepatology. 2013;**11**(10):1358-1365.e1. DOI: 10.1016/j.cgh.2013.04.028

[7] Vilgrain V, Pereira H, Assenat E, Guiu B, Ilonca AD, Pageaux GP, et al. Efficacy and safety of selective internal radiotherapy with yttrium-90 resin microspheres compared with sorafenib in locally advanced and inoperable hepatocellular carcinoma (SARAH): An open-label randomised controlled phase 3 trial. The Lancet Oncology. 2017; **18**(12):1624-1636. DOI: 10.1016/S1470-2045(17)30683-6

[8] Kallini JR, Gabr A, Salem R, Lewandowski RJ. Transarterial radioembolization with Yttrium-90 for the treatment of hepatocellular carcinoma. Advances in Therapy. 2016; **33**(5):699-714. DOI: 10.1007/s12325-016-0324-7

[9] Lewandowski RJ, Salem R. Yttrium-90 radioembolization of hepatocellular carcinoma and metastatic disease to the liver. Seminars in Interventional Radiology. 2006;**23**(1):64-72. DOI: 10.1055/s-2006-939842

[10] Miller FH, Lopes Vendrami C, Gabr A, Horowitz JM, Kelahan LC, Riaz A, et al. Evolution of radioembolization in treatment of hepatocellular carcinoma: A pictorial review. Radiographics. 2021;**41**(6): 1802-1818

[11] Kim SP, Cohalan C, Kopek N, Enger SA. A guide to ^{90}Y radioembolization and its dosimetry. Physica Medica. 2019;**68**:132-145. DOI: 10.1016/j.ejmp.2019.09.236

[12] Salem R, Lewandowski RJ, Mulcahy MF, Riaz A, Ryu RK, Ibrahim S, et al. Radioembolization for hepatocellular carcinoma using Yttrium-90 microspheres: A comprehensive report of long-term outcomes. Gastroenterology. 2010;**138**(1):52-64. DOI: 10.1053/j.gastro.2009.09.006

[13] Sato K, Lewandowski RJ, Bui JT, Omary R, Hunter RD, Kulik L, et al. Treatment of unresectable primary and metastatic liver cancer with yttrium-90 microspheres (TheraSphere): Assessment of hepatic arterial embolization. Cardiovascular and Interventional Radiology. 2006;**29**(4): 522-529. DOI: 10.1007/s00270-005-0171-4

[14] Murthy R, Xiong H, Nunez R, Cohen AC, Barron B, Szklaruk J, et al. Yttrium 90 resin microspheres for the treatment of unresectable colorectal hepatic metastases after failure of multiple chemotherapy regimens: Preliminary results. Journal of Vascular and Interventional Radiology. 2005; **16**(7):937-945. DOI: 10.1097/01.RVI.0000161142.12822.66

[15] Noussios G, Dimitriou I, Chatzis I, Katsourakis A. The main anatomic variations of the hepatic artery and their importance in surgical practice: Review of the literature. Journal of Clinical Medical Research. 2017;**9**(4):248-252. DOI: 10.14740/jocmr2902w

[16] Song SY, Chung JW, Lim HG, Park JH. Nonhepatic arteries originating from the hepatic arteries: Angiographic analysis in 250 patients. Journal of Vascular and Interventional Radiology. 2006;**17**(3):461-469. DOI: 10.1097/01.rvi.0000202718.16416.18

[17] Lewandowski RJ, Sato KT, Atassi B, Ryu RK, Nemcek AA Jr, Kulik L, et al. Radioembolization with 90Y microspheres: Angiographic and technical considerations. Cardiovascular and Interventional Radiology. 2007; **30**(4):571-592. DOI: 10.1007/s00270-007-9064-z

[18] Son MH, Ha LN, Bang MH, Bae S, Giang DT, Thinh NT, et al. Diagnostic and prognostic value of ^{99m}Tc-MAA SPECT/CT for treatment planning of ^{90}Y-resin microsphere radioembolization for hepatocellular carcinoma: Comparison with planar image. Scientific Reports. 2021;**11**(1): 3207. DOI: 10.1038/s41598-021-82887-w

[19] Villalobos A, Soliman MM, Majdalany BS, Schuster DM, Galt J, Bercu ZL, et al. Yttrium-90 radioembolization dosimetry: What trainees need to know. Seminars in Interventional Radiology. 2020;**37**(5): 543-554. DOI: 10.1055/s-0040-1720954

[20] d'Abadie P, Hesse M, Louppe A, Lhommel R, Walrand S, Jamar F. Microspheres used in liver radioembolization: From conception to clinical effects. Molecules. 2021;**26**(13): 3966. DOI: 10.3390/molecules26133966

[21] Kim YC, Kim YH, Uhm SH, Seo YS, Park EK, Oh SY, et al. Radiation safety issues in y-90 microsphere selective hepatic radioembolization therapy: Possible radiation exposure from the patients. Nuclear Medicine and Molecular Imaging. 2010;**44**(4):252-260. DOI: 10.1007/s13139-010-0047-7

[22] Vanani NB, Janardan A, Asmi N, Jha P. Post-embolization syndrome following Yttrium-90 radiation segmentectomy. Cureus. 2023;**15**(3): e35947. DOI: 10.7759/cureus.35947

[23] Riaz A, Awais R, Salem R. Side effects of yttrium-90 radioembolization. Frontiers in Oncology. 2014;**4**:198. DOI: 10.3389/fonc.2014.00198

[24] Braat MN, van Erpecum KJ, Zonnenberg BA, van den Bosch MA, Lam MG. Radioembolization-induced liver disease: A systematic review. European Journal of Gastroenterology & Hepatology. 2017;**29**(2):144-152. DOI: 10.1097/MEG.0000000000000772

[25] Badar W, Van Ha T, Zangan S, Navuluri R, Pillai A, Baker T, et al. Safety and efficacy of repeat Y90 radioembolization to the same hepatic arterial territory. The British Journal of Radiology. 2021;**94**(1119):20200752. DOI: 10.1259/bjr.20200752

[26] Lencioni R, Llovet JM. Modified RECIST (mRECIST) assessment for hepatocellular carcinoma. Seminars in Liver Disease. 2010;**30**(1):52-60. DOI: 10.1055/s-0030-1247132

[27] Cunha GM, Sirlin CB, Fowler KJ. Imaging diagnosis of hepatocellular carcinoma: LI-RADS. Chinese Clinical Oncology. 2021;**10**(1):3. DOI: 10.21037/cco-20-107

[28] Lewandowski RJ, Gabr A, Abouchaleh N, Ali R, Al Asadi A, Mora RA, et al. Radiation segmentectomy: Potential curative therapy for early hepatocellular carcinoma. Radiology. 2018;**287**(3):1050-1058. DOI: 10.1148/radiol.2018171768

[29] Salem R, Johnson GE, Kim E, Riaz A, Bishay V, Boucher E, et al. Yttrium-90 radioembolization for the treatment of solitary, unresectable HCC: The LEGACY Study. Hepatology. 2021;**74**(5):2342-2352. DOI: 10.1002/hep.31819

[30] Gaba RC, Lewandowski RJ, Kulik LM, Riaz A, Ibrahim SM, Mulcahy MF, et al. Radiation lobectomy: Preliminary findings of hepatic volumetric response to lobar yttrium-90 radioembolization. Annals of Surgical Oncology. 2009;**16**(6):1587-1596. DOI: 10.1245/s10434-009-0454-0

[31] Teo JY, Goh BK. Contra-lateral liver lobe hypertrophy after unilobar Y90 radioembolization: An alternative to portal vein embolization? World Journal of Gastroenterology. 2015;**21**(11):3170-3173. DOI: 10.3748/wjg.v21.i11.3170

Chapter 5

The Pathophysiology of Hepatic Encephalopathy at the Level of Gut-Liver-Brain Axis: The Role of Resident Innate Immune Cells

Ali Sepehrinezhad and Ali Shahbazi

Abstract

Hepatic encephalopathy (HE) reflects a wide spectrum of frequent and complex neurological complications that are associated with advanced liver diseases. It significantly impacts the quality of life and daily activities of those affected. Despite many investigations, the precise pathophysiology of HE is still under discussion. One contributing factor believed to be responsible for HE is the accumulation of neurotoxic substances in the brain such as ammonia, mercaptans, short-chain fatty acids, and lipopolysaccharides, originating from the dysfunctional liver. Strong data, however, suggests that HE is a complex symptom, and inflammation interacts synergistically with ammonia to worsen gliopathy and neuronal destruction. Recent data suggests that HE might come from the intestines. Increased activity of gut innate immune cells, especially macrophages and dendritic cells, can initiate inflammatory signals from the gut to systemic circulation, liver tissue, and finally the central nervous system. In this chapter, all inflammatory mechanisms at the levels of the gut-liver-brain axis following cirrhosis and HE are presented in detail. The chapter highlights the role of intestinal innate immune cells, liver Kupffer cells, and brain microglia in cirrhosis and the progression of HE.

Keywords: cirrhosis, hepatic encephalopathy, gut-liver-brain axis, innate immune cells, intestinal macrophages, Kupffer cells, microglia

1. Introduction

Hepatic encephalopathy (HE) is a frequent neurological disorder and a serious consequence of advanced liver disease, acute liver failure, or portal-systemic shunting. HE is defined as a wide range of neuropsychiatric disturbances, including changes in personality, a shortened attention span, intellectual disability, cognitive impairment, alterations in sleep patterns, delirium, asterixis, episodic confusion, seizures, decreased level of consciousness, and even coma [1–3]. Three varieties of HE

IntechOpen

are distinguished based on the underlying cause. Type A refers to brain dysfunction that arises as a result of acute liver failure. Type B is observed in cases where there is portosystemic shunting without liver insufficiency, and type C as a consequence of liver cirrhosis [3, 4]. According to the West Haven Criteria (WHC), HE is categorized into grades I to IV, ranging from a lack of attention (grade I) to coma (grade IV). Based on the severity of manifestations, the International Society of Hepatic Encephalopathy and Nitrogen Metabolism (ISHEN) classifies HE into two categories: covert HE (CHE) and overt HE (OHE). CHE refers to minimal HE (MHE) and grade I HE, which are characterized by neuropsychological alterations without clinical evidence of mental changes. On the other hand, OHE displays severe neurological manifestations [3, 5]. The exact mechanism behind brain dysfunction in patients with liver diseases is complex and not yet fully revealed. However, it has been agreed that ammonia plays a key role. It mainly originates from the degradation of nitrogen-containing compounds by the intestinal microbiome, as well as the hydrolysis of glutamine by gut glutaminase, which is then transported into the portal circulation. A large portion of circulating ammonia is metabolized in the urea cycle by intact hepatocytes and subsequently excreted by the kidneys as urea [6]. In patients with liver insufficiency, the injured hepatocytes are no longer able to effectively detoxify ammonia from the blood. Subsequently, the level of circulatory ammonia is increased, which can result in a condition called hyperammonemia. Increased levels of ammonia in systemic circulation can cause detrimental effects on the central nervous system (CNS) through various pathways [6, 7]. Findings from numerous animal and clinical studies have indicated that inflammation, synergistically with ammonia, can potentially link to the development of HE [8–12]. Recently, there has been a growing focus among researchers on finding out the pathogenesis of brain dysfunction that occurs following liver diseases in organs beyond the liver and CNS [13]. Evidence indicates a correlation between alteration of gut microbiota composition (gut dysbiosis) and its associated by-products with conditions such as intestinal and liver inflammation, systemic inflammation, hyperammonemia, and neuroinflammation in liver diseases and HE [14–17]. The gut, liver, and brain have some strong associations. The portal system allows a considerable part of the blood that passes through the gastrointestinal tract and many gut-active metabolites to reach the liver parenchyma. Similarly, the liver can influence intestine processes by synthesizing and secreting bile acids. Furthermore, both the gut and the liver can control various cerebral processes via their metabolites and immune systems. Moreover, through a cascade of humoral, neuroendocrine, immunological, neural, and metabolic signals, the brain can alter the activities of the liver and intestines [18–20]. The gut-liver-brain axis is a fascinating concept that involves a complex and multidirectional communication pathway linking the gastrointestinal tract, hepatic system, and CNS. In this axis, the brain influences the activity of gut and hepatic innate immune cells, while the liver and intestine regulate mental processes through gut microbiota and immune interactions [21, 22]. Recent reports indicate that impairment of the gut-liver-brain axis may play a role in the pathophysiology of liver diseases and HE [23–25]. It has been reported that the components of the innate immune system are considered the main communication route between the gut, liver, and brain. Innate immune cells found in the enteric, hepatic, and central nervous systems may mediate complicated connections between these organs. Researchers would benefit from an accurate understanding of the inflammatory signals emanating from residual innate immune cells and their impact on the gut-liver-brain axis in advanced liver disease and HE.

2. Intestinal macrophages and dendritic cells produce gut inflammatory signals

Gut macrophages (Mϕ), like other tissue Mϕ, originate from pluripotent bone marrow stem cells that develop into circulatory monocytes in the presence of interleukin (IL)-1, IL-3, IL-6, and granulocyte-macrophage colony-stimulating factor (GM-CSF). Circulatory monocytes eventually extravasate into the intestinal lamina proparia, submucosal, and myentric plexus, where they come into contact with mucosal epithelium, luminal contents, and the enteric nervous system (ENS) [26, 27]. C-C motif chemokine receptor 2 (CCR2) signaling is totally required for blood monocyte penetration into the gut [28]. In mice, newly recruited monocytes are identified by the expression of profibrotic Ly6C and C-X3-C motif chemokine receptor 1 (CX3CR1), whereas mature resident intestinal Mϕ is identified by the expression of CD14, CD11b, MHCII, CX3CR1, and CD64 markers [28]. Furthermore, mediators, such as colony-stimulating factor 1 (CSF-1), transforming growth factor beta (TGFβ), IL-10, and CX3CR1, aid in the differentiation of monocytes into mature Mϕ [28–31]. Intestinal Mϕ phagocytize pathogens as they express high levels of phagocytic markers such as Cd36, Gas6, Mertk, Axl, Itgav, Mrc1, Itgb5, Cd81, and C1qa-c [32]. They also express the efferocytosis receptor αvβ5, which facilitates the scavenging of apoptotic epithelial cells, hence maintaining the integrity of the mucosal epithelial barrier [33, 34]. The intestinal barrier and mucosal integrity are safeguarded by mediators produced by gut Mϕ, such as hepatocyte growth factor (HGF), Wnt signaling elements, IL-10, and prostaglandin E2 (PGE2) and their balloon-like protrusions [35–38]. Additionally, intestinal Mϕ receives components of the luminal side through their projection processes into the mucosal layer. They play an important role in the presentation of antigens to dendritic cells (DCs) in the lamina proparia and the activation of T cells [39]. Gut Mϕ also interacts with both neural cells in ENS and enteric smooth muscle cells through the bone morphogenetic protein 2 (BMP2) and transient receptor potential cation channel subfamily V Member 4 (TRPV4)-PGE2-E-prostanoid receptor 1 or 3 (EP1/3) pathways, respectively [40, 41]. Colony stimulating factor 1 (CSF-1) is also secreted by ENS neurons, and it controls macrophage activity by binding to its membrane-bound CSF-1 receptors [42]. These multidirectional pathways allow Mϕ to regulate intestinal motility.

The homeostasis of the gut environment is maintained by an integrated epithelial mucosal barrier and intact tight junctions. Patients with cirrhosis and HE have been shown to have gut dysbiosis and a change in the composition of their gut microbiome from normal flora to pathogenic species such as *Streptococcus salivarius*, Proteobacteria, and Enterobacteriaceae [17, 43, 44]. Gut microbiota alteration was also revealed in several experimental animal models of liver disease and HE (**Table 1**) [63–67]. In addition, these patients had small bowel bacterial overgrowth, as determined by Qin et al. in a quantitative metagenomics analysis, which found differences in 75,245 genes between healthy people and cirrhotic patients [68].

Study	Findings (Intestinal tissue)	References
Wang et al. (2017)	⇧Intestinal permeability (Evans blue), ⇧mucosal barrier damage, ⇧alpha1-antitrypsin, ⇧calprotectin (neutrophil infiltration), ⇩claudin-1, ⇩claudin-6, ⇩occludin, ⇧TLR4, ⇧TLR9 (CCL4 rats)	[45]
Wang et al. (2020)	⇩Occludin, ⇩ZO-1, ⇧dysbiosis (CCL4 mice)	[46]

Study	Findings (Intestinal tissue)	References
Zhou et al. 2014	⇩Occludin, ⇧mucosal injury, ⇧D-lactate and diamine oxidase (serum markers of intestinal barrier disruption) (BDL rats)	[47]
Wang et al. (2021)	⇩Villus height and width, ⇩crypt depth, ⇩Occludin, ⇩ZO-1, ⇩claudin-1 (CCL4 mice)	[48]
Luyer et al. (2004)	⇧Bacterial translocation (BDL rats)	[49]
Liu et al. (2020)	⇧Dysbiosis, (CCL4 mice) ⇧Bacteroidaceae, ⇧Porphyromonadaceae, ⇧Marinillabiliaceae, ⇧Chloroplast, ⇧Methylobacteriaceae, ⇧Enterobacteriaceae, ⇧Streptococcaceae, ⇧Lactobacillaceae (small intestine)	[14]
	⇧Marinillabiliaceae, ⇧Prevotellaceae, ⇧Bacteroidales Incertae Sedis, ⇧Flammeovirgaceae, ⇧Streptococcaceae, ⇧Enterobacteriaceae, ⇧Methylobacteriaceae (colon)	
Palma et al. (2007)	⇧Bacterial translocation (CCL4 rats)	[50]
Lei et al. (2022)	⇩Occludin, ⇩claudin-1, ⇩ZO-1, ⇧NF-κB, (BDL rats)	[51]
Fu et al. (2022)	⇩Occludin mRNA and protein, ⇩ZO-1 mRNA and protein, ⇩claudin-1 mRNA and protein, ⇧endotoxemia (⇧LPS and ⇧MIP-1 in serum), ⇧dysbiosis (CCL4 mice)	[52]
Sánchez et al. (2014)	⇧Bacterial translocation (CCL4 rats)	[53]
Cabrera-Rubio et al. (2019)	⇧Gut dysbiosis (⇧Akkermansia, ⇧Bacteroides, ⇧Ruminococcaceae, ⇧Prevotella, ⇩*Faecalibacterium prausnitzii*) (BDL mice)	[54]
Zhao et al. (2021)	⇩Claudin-1 mRNA, ⇧HMGB1 mRNA, ⇧TLR4 mRNA, ⇧MyD88 mRNA, ⇧NF-kβ mRNA (CCL4 rats)	[55]
Safari et al. (2023)	⇩Occludin, ⇩claudin-1, ⇩farnesoid X receptor (FXR), ⇧claudin-2 (BDL rats)	[56]
Assimakopoulos et al. (2003)	⇧Endotoxemia, ⇧lipid peroxidation, ⇧protein oxidation, ⇧oxidized glutathione, ⇩glutathione (BDL rats)	[57]
Chen et al. (2014)	⇧Gut dysbiosis (patients with cirrhosis)	[58]
Assimakopoulos et al. (2015)	⇧Endotoxemia, ⇩mitotic cell count, ⇧apoptosis, ⇧lipid peroxidation, (patients with cirrhosis)	[59]
Chen et al. (2011)	⇧Gut dysbiosis (⇧Proteobacteria, ⇧Fusobacteria, ⇩Bacteroidetes) (patients with cirrhosis)	[60]
Du Plessis et al. (2013)	⇧LPS (serum), ⇧$CD33^+$-$CD14^+$-Trem-1^+Mϕ, ⇧iNOS, ⇧NO, ⇧Claudin-2, ⇧intestinal barrier (patients with cirrhosis)	[61]
Pascual et al. (2003)	⇧Lactulose/mannitol ratio (marker of intestinal permeability) (patients with cirrhosis)	[62]

Table 1.
Main intestinal changes following cirrhosis and HE.

Cirrhosis-related gut dysbiosis alters intestinal barrier permeability and epithelial tight junctions through the induction of oxidative stress, immune cell infiltration, a decrease in short-chain fatty acids, and a loss in the capacity of epithelial stem cells to self-renew [59, 67, 69, 70]. Portal hypertension also impairs the intestinal barrier via perturbation of intestinal circulation and cellular hypoxia in cirrhosis [71, 72]. In cirrhosis and liver disease, decrease in expression of some intestinal antimicrobial molecules, such as α-defensin5, α-defensin6, RegIII, and β-defensin 1, may exacerbate dysbiosis and bacterial translocation [73–76]. In both rat models of acute liver failure and cirrhosis, a decrease in the expression of several intestine antimicrobial peptides was shown [77, 78]. In cirrhosis, bacterial translocation and endotoxin products, such as flagellin, peptidoglycan, lipopolysaccharide (LPS), bacterial DNA, and pathogen-associated molecular pattern molecules (PAMPs), were able to enter the lamina propria and portal circulation due to the compromised intestinal barrier [79, 80]. These endotoxins and false metabolites stimulate Mϕ and DCs in Peyer's patches of the lamina propria. Activated Mϕ synthetize and secrete pro-inflammatory cytokines such as IL-1, IL-18, TGF-β, IL-6, interferon gamma (IFNγ), IL-1β, nitric oxide (NO), and tumor necrosis factor alpha (TNFα) (**Figure 1**). These metabolites also increase the phagocytosis capacity of DCs. Increasing levels of intestinal pro-inflammatory cytokines injure the mucosal epithelial barrier and enhance neutrophil infiltration into the lamina propria. An electron microscopy analysis of biopsy samples from the duodenum revealed that patients with cirrhosis had an impaired intestinal barrier due to activated gut Mϕ and production of IL-6 and NO [61]. Fecal analysis in patients with acute decompensating cirrhosis indicated an increase in intestinal pro-inflammatory cytokines that were correlated with intestinal barrier disruption [81]. Furthermore, an increase in serum levels of LPS was associated with a decrease in the expression of intestinal tight junction proteins (i.e., occludin and claudin-1) in

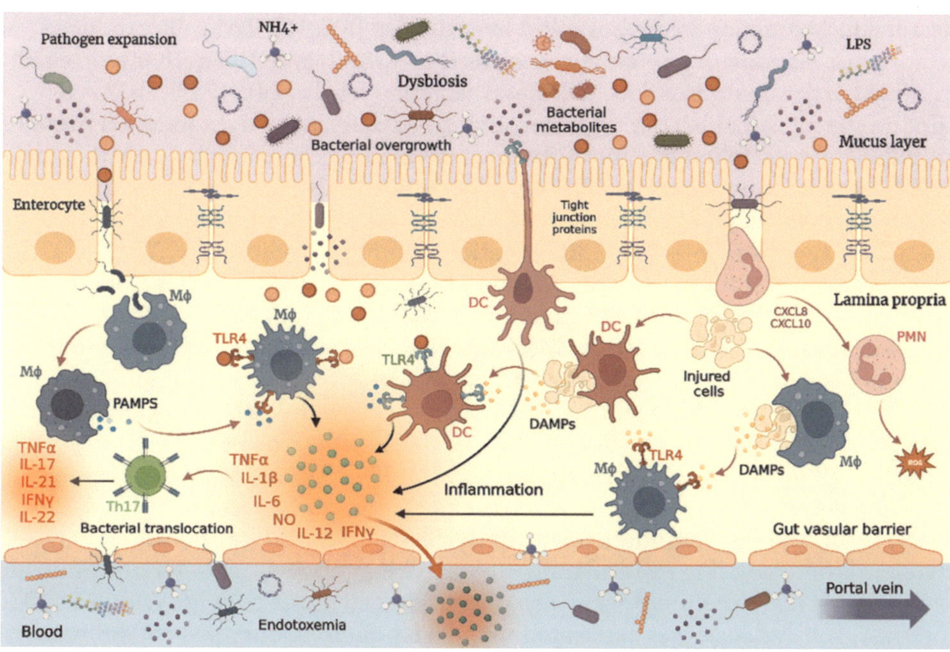

Figure 1.
Gut dysbiosis and intestinal inflammation in pathophysiology of cirrhosis and HE, highlighting the role of intestinal macrophages and dendritic cells. CXCL8, C-X-C motif chemokine ligand 8; CXCL10, C-X-C motif chemokine ligand 10; DAMPs, damage-associated molecular pattern molecules; DC, dendritic cell; IFNγ, interferon gamma; IL-1β, Interleukin-1 beta; IL-6, Interleukin-6; IL-17, Interleukin-17; IL-21, Interleukin-21; IL-22, Interleukin-22; LPS, lipopolysaccharide; Mϕ, macrophages; NH_4^+, ammonia; NO, nitric oxide; PAMPs, pathogen-associated molecular patterns; PMN, polymorphonuclear; ROS, reactive oxygen species; TLR4, toll-like receptor 4; TNFα, tumor necrosis factor alpha. Created with BioRender.com.

patients with cirrhosis [82]. IL-6 and TNFα can initiate downstream inflammatory signals by activating the nuclear factor kappa-light-chain-enhancer of activated B cells (NF-kβ) [83–87]. The number of NO-releasing duodenal $CD33^+$-$CD14^+$-Trem-1^+ Mϕ increased in cirrhosis. Additionally, these patients had higher levels of blood pro-inflammatory cytokines and circulatory LPS, as well as overexpressed claudin-2, a permeable tight protein, in the duodenum [61]. Injured epithelial cells and activated Mϕ release damage-associated molecular patterns (DAMPs). These DAMPs, along with PAMPs, have the ability to activate pattern recognition receptors (PRRs), particularly toll-like receptors (TLRs) that are found in intestinal Mϕ and DCs [88, 89]. Among the TLR family, TLR1, TLR2, TLR4, TLR5, and TLR6 are known to localize on the cell membrane and recognize various pathogen membrane elements. On the other hand, intracellular TLR3, TLR7, TLR8, and TLR9 are able to detect nucleic acids [90]. LPS derived from altered microbiota triggers an inflammatory signaling pathway through TLR4 in Mϕ (**Figure 1**). This pathway involves the activation of signaling proteins, including TRAM, TRIF, RIP1, TRF3, or TRAF6, which subsequently lead to the overexpression of MAPK and NF-kβ proteins [91, 92]. The majority of PAMPs can trigger PRRs, predominantly TLR2 and TLR4, on DCs. This mediates the migration of DCs to mesenteric lymph nodes, where they subsequently differentiate the naïve T cells into Th1, Th2, and inflammatory effector T cells. Activated DCs by PAMPs-TLR also present their antigens to $CD4^+$ T cells through the major histocompatibility complex II and T cell receptor interaction. Additionally, these activated DCs secrete pro-inflammatory cytokines that further activate $CD4^+$ T cells [84, 88, 93]. Increased Th1 cell numbers and an imbalanced Th17/Treg ratio have been shown to worsen intestinal inflammation in cirrhosis and liver disease [67, 94]. Th1 cells produced several pro-inflammatory cytokines, such as IFN-γ, IL-2, and TNFα, that worsened intestinal barrier disruption [95, 96]. Basal secreting levels of IL-17 by Th17 cells maintain the intestinal barrier by increasing the expression of tight junction proteins [97, 98]. However, following gut dysbiosis, activated Mϕ and DCs by PAMPs and DAMPs increase the number of Th17 cells by secreting IL-23, IL-6, and IL-1β. A number of powerful pro-inflammatory cytokines are produced by activated Th17 cells, which aggravate intestinal inflammation [99–102]. Additionally, Th17-derived cytokines stimulate the production of neutrophil chemotaxis factors such as IL-8, C-X-C motif chemokine ligand 8 (CXCL8), GM-CSF, and C-X-C motif chemokine ligand 10 (CXCL10) by Mϕ, epithelial cells, and DCs [103]. Moreover, cytokines produced by Th17 cells prevent naive T cells from differentiating into Treg cells. Treg cells produce and secrete anti-inflammatory cytokines in response to activated DCs [104].

Finally, all pro-inflammatory cytokines, chemokines, PAMPs, DAMPs, and gut microbiome-derived ammonia can reach the portal circulation and result in systemic inflammation and hyperammonemia. Gut dysbiosis, bacterial translocation, and elevated levels of circulating pro-inflammatory cytokines, as well as bacterial metabolites (i.e. methanol and threonine) were also observed in cirrhosis patients with HE [105]. Moreover, gut dysbiosis was associated with levels of circulatory pro-inflammatory cytokines, and circulatory bacterial products were positively associated with HE [105]. Likewise, elevated serum levels of pro-inflammatory cytokines, including IFN-γ, IL-1β, and IL-6, were also correlated with grade of HE in patients with cirrhosis [106]. In cirrhosis patients with HE, the systemic inflammatory response score was also positively correlated with the grade of HE [107]. Furthermore, systemic inflammatory response and hyperammonemia were also reported in acute-on-chronic liver failure (ACLF) and HE patients. Also, in these patients, blood ammonia was correlated with grade of HE and mortality rate [108]. Furthermore, cirrhotic patients with history of previous HE presented higher levels of circulatory IL-6, IL-2, IL-1β, TNFα, and endotoxins [43]. Gut microbiome alteration was also correlated with systemic inflammation in these patients [43]. Increase the number of Th17 cells and reduce the population of Treg, resulting in decrease the Treg/Th17 ratio shown in the blood circulation of cirrhosis patients due to hepatitis C virus [94]. Soluble sCD163 is a good marker that represents monocyte expansion and macrophage activation [109]. The circulatory level of this peptide was significantly raised in cirrhotic patients with ACLF [110]. An increase in serum inflammatory mediators was also revealed in carbon tetrachloride (CCL4)-induced cirrhosis and HE in rats [106]. Furthermore, our group indicated that the levels of pro-inflammatory mediators and ammonia are increased in thioacetamide-induced HE mice [23]. Increased concentrations of pro-inflammatory cytokines, active monocytes, T helper $CD34^+$ cells, and bacterial DNA were seen in circulation of CCL4-induced cirrhosis rats [85]. Moreover, the number of T helper $CD34^+$ cells and monocytes as well as elevated levels of bacterial DNA were demonstrated in the mesenteric lymph nodes of these rats [85].

3. Activated Kupffer cells exacerbate hepatocyte injury and systemic inflammation

Active bacterial metabolites and products, DAMPs, gut-derived pro-inflammatory cytokines, ammonia, and activated immune cells finally reach the liver through the portal vein and are directly exposed to other types of body-resident Mϕ named Kupffer cells (KCs) [111]. They are localized to hepatic sinusoidal endothelial cells and have a great role in scavenging circulatory pathogenic agents (**Figure 2**). The KCs are amoeboid-shaped cells with several processes, including microvilli, lamellipodia, and pseudopodia, that let them move around and endocytosis pathogens, apoptotic cells, and endotoxins [112]. The liver KCs originate from the embryonic yolk sac and have self-renewing properties [113, 114]. However, it has been shown that bone marrow-derived circulatory monocytes can be differentiated into KCs [115]. The KCs are functionally divided into two distinct types: M1 (pro-inflammatory classically activated KCs) and M2 (anti-inflammatory alternatively activated KCs). M1 KCs are activated in response to LPS, bacterial DNA, and pathogens, as well as pro-inflammatory mediators, resulting in the induction of oxidative stress and the production of pro-inflammatory cytokines. On the other hand, M2 KCs are triggered in response to IL-10, IL-13, and IL4, which lead to the secretion of anti-inflammatory cytokines [116–118]. KCs express several surface receptors that distinguish them from other cell types in the liver parenchyma. These molecules include CD68, CD14, and TLR4 in humans and CD11b, CD68, F4/80, CD163, CLEC4F, TIM4, TLR4, TLR9, and CRIg in rodents [119].

In liver cirrhosis, hepatocyte injury produces a substantial amount of DAMPs such as apoptotic bodies, ATP, high mobility group protein B1 (HMGB1), ATP, and DNA in the perisinusoidal space (space of Disse), where hepatic stellate cells (HSCs) are located (**Figure 2**) [120–122]. These agents, along with PAMPs and other gut-derived metabolites, activate HSCs to secrete monocyte and neutrophil chemotactic agents, such as chemokine (C-C motif) ligand 2, as well as activate KCs [123]. Moreover, KCs, through some mediators such as TGFβ, CCL2, CCL3, and CCL5 activate HSCs [124]. The HSCs progress liver fibrosis through a signaling pathway dependent on TGFβ, NLRP3 inflammasome-Caspase1-IL1β, and WNT/β-catenin [125–127]. Like intestinal

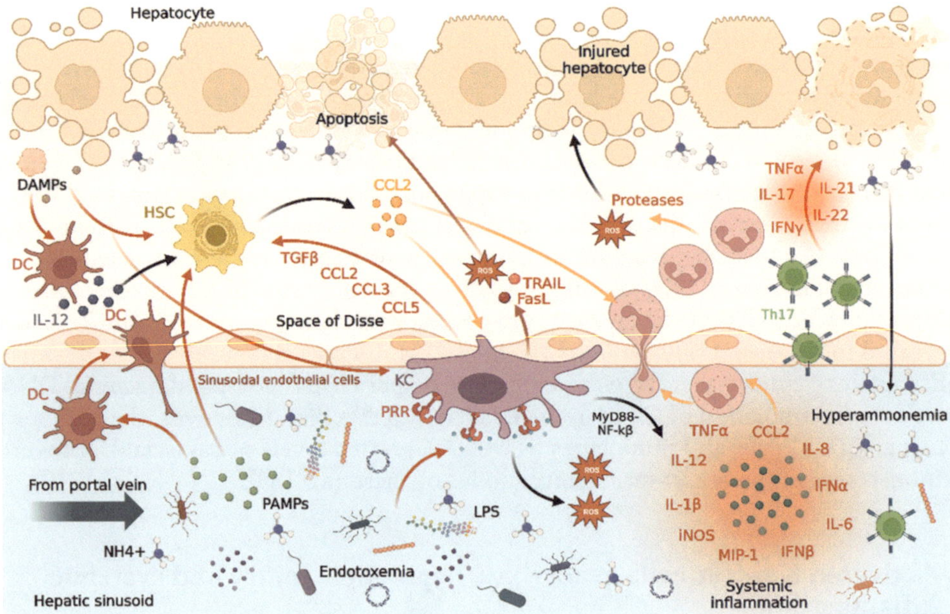

Figure 2.
Activated Kupffer cells induce liver inflammation and exacerbate systemic inflammation in cirrhosis and HE. DAMPs, damage-associated molecular pattern molecules; CCL2, C-C motif chemokine ligand 2; CCL3, C-C motif chemokine ligand 2; CCL5, C-C motif chemokine ligand 5; DC, dendritic cell; FasL, Fas ligand; HSC, hepatic stellate cell; iNOS, inducible nitric oxide synthases; IFNα, interferon alpha; IFNβ, interferon beta; IFNγ, interferon gamma; IL-1β, Interleukin-1 beta; IL-6, Interleukin-6; IL-8, Interleukin-8; IL-12, Interleukin-12; IL-17, Interleukin-17; IL-21, Interleukin-21; IL-22, Interleukin-22; KC, Kupffer cell; LPS, lipopolysaccharide; MIP-1, macrophage inflammatory protein-1; NF-kβ, nuclear factor kappa-light-chain-enhancer of activated B cells; NH_4^+, ammonia; PAMPs, pathogen-associated molecular patterns; PRR, pattern recognition receptors; ROS, reactive oxygen species; TGFβ, transforming growth factor-β; TNFα, tumor necrosis factor alpha; TRAIL, TNF-related apoptosis-inducing ligand. Created with BioRender.com

Mϕ, KCs express PRRs on their surface, including TLR, RIG-like receptors, C-type lectin receptors (CLR), and nucleotide-binding oligomerization domain (NOD)-like receptors that recognize DAMPs and PAMPs [128–130]. For instance, activation of TLR4 in response to circulatory LPS through activation of myeloid differentiation factor 88 and overexpression of NF-kβ induces the production of pro-inflammatory cytokines such as IL-1β, IL-6, IL-8, TNFα, intercellular adhesion molecule 1 (ICAM-1) and vascular cell adhesion molecule 1 (VCAM-1) [129, 131–133]. Moreover, activation of intracellular TLR3 in response to viral RNA through activation of TRIF and IRF3 produces IFNα and IFNβ in KCs [134]. In response to elevated levels of sinusoidal DAMPs and PAMPs, KCs are activated and release pro-inflammatory mediators (i.e. IL-12, IL-1β, iNOS, CCL2, and MIP-1) and induce oxidative stress in the liver parenchyma [118, 135]. Activated KCs also secrete Fas ligand (FasL), tumor necrosis factor-related apoptosis-inducing ligand (TRAIL), and TNFα that trigger hepatocyte apoptosis [136]. Triggered KCs also exacerbate the recruitment of neutrophils and circulatory monocytes through production of several chemoattractant chemokines, such as CXCL1, CXCL2, CXCL8, CCL1, CCL2, and CCL25 in cirrhosis [137]. DCs are also triggered by activated KCs, DAMPs, PAMPs, and liver inflammation. According to function and surface receptors, five subsets of DCs are present in the nonlymphoid tissue of humans and mice. This includes Langerhans DCs ($CD207^+$ and $CD14^-$, human), $CD11b^+$ cells ($CD207^-$, $CD14^+$, $BDCA1^+$ and $CD11c^{high}$, human), $CD8\alpha^+$-like conventional cells ($CD207^-$, $CD14^-$, $CD1a^+$, $BDCA3^+$ and $CD11c^{high}$, human), monocyte-derived cells ($Lyc6C^+$, $MAC3^+$, $CD11b^+$ and $CD11c^+$, mouse), and plasmacytoid DCs ($BDCA3^+$, CD11c-, human) [138–141]. Two subtypes, including monocyte-derived and plasmacytoid DCs, are implicated in liver cirrhosis [142, 143]. The monocyte-derived DCs express TLR4, TLR8, and NOD-like receptors, while the plasmacytoid DCs express TLR1, TLR7, and TLR9 in both humans and mice [140, 144, 145]. In response to KCs-derived chemokines and liver inflammation, DCs recruit to the liver parenchyma. Liver DCs also express PRRs that mediate their responses to DAMPs and PAMPs. Activated DCs may trigger HSCs and $CD8^+$ T cells through the secretion of IL-12 and programmed death ligand 1 (PD-L1), respectively [146, 147]. DCs also express MHC I and II peptides, which interact with CD8+ and CD4+ receptors and result in the activation of T cells. Moreover, activated DCs can trigger the differentiation of T cells through the production of IL-12 and IFNγ [148]. Severe infiltration of monocyte-derived and plasmacytoid DCs in the liver parenchyma along with increased production of IFNα have been reported in cirrhotic patients with ACLF [142]. In CCL4-induced cirrhosis and HE mouse models, liver inflammation along with increase in the number of $CD11c^+$-$MHCII^{high}$-$CD11b^+$ DCs have been shown in liver tissue [149]. Activated KCs and DCs have an impact on T cell activity. An increase in the infiltration of inflammatory Th17 cells in the liver parenchyma of patients with chronic hepatitis C has been shown [150]. Moreover, the recruitment of Th17 cells in liver tissue was correlated with grade of liver inflammation [150]. Likewise, the population of Th17 cells is increased in blood and liver tissue of patients with chronic hepatitis B and cirrhosis. Also, raise in the infiltration of Th17 cells into the liver parenchyma and an elevated level of IL-17 were associated with the severity of the disease and grade of liver fibrosis [151]. Furthermore, an increase in the Th17/Treg ratio along with overexpression of NF-kβ, TNFα, IL-1β, and IL-6 was revealed in patients with hepatitis B and cirrhosis [152]. In cirrhotic rats, an increase in the population of $CD3^+$ T cells, T helper cells ($CD4^+$-$CD8^-$), and $CD134^+$ T cells were observed in hepatic lymph nodes [85]. Moreover, overexpression of IL-17 mRNA and protein was demonstrated in the liver tissue of bile duct ligation (BDL) rats as a model of chronic liver failure-induced HE [153]. In cirrhosis, the detoxification of ammonia, as well as endogenous agents, PAMPs, and DAMPs by injured hepatocytes is compromised, leading to liver inflammation (**Table 2**) and elevated levels of these compounds in the systemic circulation. Moreover, pro-inflammatory cytokines and chemokines produced by activated KCs, HSCs, DCs, and infiltrating neutrophils can be released into systemic blood flow and eventually make their way to the brain.

Study	Findings (Liver tissue)	References
Luckey et al. (2001)	⇧TNFα mRNA, ⇧IL-6 mRNA, ⇧IL-1β mRNA, ⇧cyclooxygenase 2 mRNA, ⇧CD14 mRNA, ⇧I kappa B alpha transcription (in activated Kupffer cells of CCL4 rats)	[154]
Aoyama et al. (2010)	⇧CX3CR1 mRNA, ⇧CX3CL1 mRNA, ⇧MIP-1α mRNA, ⇧MIP-1β mRNA, ⇧CD68 mRNA, ⇧IL-10, ⇧arginase-1 mRNA, ⇧TIMP Metallopeptidase Inhibitor 1 (TIMP-1) mRNA, ⇧alpha-smooth muscle actin (α-SMA; a marker for visualizing the activated hepatic stellate cells) (CCL4 mice)	[155]
Dhanda et al. (2018)	⇧IL-6 mRNA and protein, ⇧TNFα mRNA and protein, ⇧MCP-1 mRNA and protein (BDL rats)	[156]
Tung et al. (2015)	⇧Cells infiltration, ⇧bridging necrosis (BDL rats)	[157]
Kang et al. (2014)	⇧Swollen and necrotic hepatocytes (CCL4 mice)	[158]

Study	Findings (Liver tissue)	References
Moleset al. (2014)	⇧α-SMA mRNA and protein, ⇧CXCL2 mRNA, ⇧TNFα mRNA, ⇧S100 calcium-binding protein A9 (S100a9) mRNA, ⇧neutrophil recruitment (CCL4 mice)	[159]
Altaş et al. (2011)	⇧Malondialdehyde, ⇧hepatocyte degeneration, ⇧vacuolization, ⇧ hepatocytes necrosis (CCL4 rats)	[160]
Tag et al. (2015)	⇧Portal fibrosis, ⇧perisinusoidal fibrosis, ⇧α-SMA, ⇧vimentin, ⇧CD45, ⇧infiltration of leukocytes (BDL rats)	[161]
Canbay et al. (2004)	⇧CXCL1 mRNA, ⇧MIP-2 mRNA, ⇧TGFβ mRNA, ⇧collagen 1 (BDL mice)	[162]
Trebicka et al. (2010)	⇧collagen accumulation, ⇧α-SMA, ⇧myofibroblasts accumulation, ⇧TGFβ1 mRNA, ⇧Platelet-derived growth factor (PDGF) mRNA, ⇧Connective tissue growth factor (CTGF) mRNA, ⇧Matrix Metallopeptidase 2 (MMP2) mRNA, ⇧inflammation (BDL rats)	[163]
Gobejishvili et al. (2013)	⇧Apoptosis, ⇧TNFα mRNA, ⇧TGFβ1, ⇧αSMA mRNA and reactivity (BDL rats)	[164]
Weng et al. (2018)	⇧Infiltration of inflammatory cells, ⇧biliary necrosis, ⇧TNFα mRNA, ⇧IL-6 mRNA, ⇧NF-kβ mRNA (BDL mice)	[165]
Gehring et al. (2005)	⇧periportal inflammation, ⇧bile duct proliferation, ⇧hepatocyte necrosis, ⇧neutrophil recruitment (BDL mice)	[166]
Alric et al. (2000)	⇧ED-1 (activated KCs and Mϕ marker), ⇧ED-2 (activated KCS marker) (CCL4 rats)	[167]
Nagano et al. (1999)	⇧IL-5 mRNA, ⇧-6 mRNA, ⇧IL-12 mRNA (primary biliary cirrhosis patients)	[168]
Holland-Fischer et al. (2015)	⇧Serum soluble CD163 (KCs activation), ⇧serum lipopolysaccharide binding protein (Cirrhosis patients)	[169]
de Lalla et al. (2004)	⇧IFNγ, ⇧IL-4, ⇧IL-13, ⇧CD1d + cells (infiltrating antigen presenting cells marker), ⇧periportal inflammation, ⇧fibrosis (cirrhosis patients with hepatitis B)	[170]
Napoli et al. (1996)	⇧IL-2 mRNA, ⇧IFNγ mRNA, ⇩IL-10 mRNA (Cirrhosis patients)	[171]
Farinati et al. (2006)	⇧IL-1β mRNA, ⇧c-Myc mRNA, ⇧8-hydroxydeoxyguanosine (a product of DAN oxidative damage) (patients with cirrhosis)	[172]
Li et al. (2015)	⇧Casphase 3, ⇧apoptosis, ⇧pigmented hepatocytes, ⇧ductular reaction, ⇧canalicular bilirubinostasis, ⇧TGFβ, ⇧IL-10 (patients with cirrhosis)	[173]
Chuang et al. (2006)	⇧CD56+ cells (natural killer cells) (patients with primary biliary cirrhosis)	[174]

Table 2.
Significant hepatic alterations following cirrhosis and HE.

4. Activated brain microglia induce neuroinflammation

One subset of cerebral glial cells, known as brain microglia, makes up approximately 10–15% of the cells in the brain parenchyma. As resident macrophage cells, microglia differentiate from progenitors in the yolk sac and develop through CSF-1 and IL-34 signaling. During the development of the CNS, microglia have a crucial role in programmed cell death, neurogenesis, phagocytosis of neuronal cells, reforming synapses, and survival of neural progenitor cells [175–177]. Under normal conditions, microglia scavenge brain parenchyma from dead cells, apoptotic neurons, and misfolding proteins (*via* phagocytosis), maintain the activity of other brain cells (i.e. astrocytes, oligodendrocytes, and neurons) through extracellular signaling molecules, remodeling false synapses and presenting antigens in the CNS [178–181]. Basically, the central nervous system is protected from circulatory neurotoxic substances through a well-organized and intact blood-brain barrier (BBB). The BBB is a multilayer semi-permeable structure that consists of capillary single-layer endothelial cells, the basement membrane, pericytes, and the astrocyte end-feet [182, 183]. This barrier is restricted, and only lipophilic molecules (MW 500 Da) are permitted to passively cross through this structure. Moreover, carrier-mediated transport facilitates the transportation of glucose and amino acids. Other limit transport systems (i.e. restricted paracellular pathway, transcytosis transport) mediated the entry of hydrated ions, low-density lipoprotein, iron, and insulin-like growth factor into the brain tissue [17, 183]. Transport across the BBB is constrained by several proteins, such as claudin-5 and occludin, zonula occludens-1 (ZO-1), and junctional adhesion molecules between endothelial cells (paracellular pathway). Systemic inflammation and injuries negatively affect tight junction structure and functions, resulting in disruption of the integrity of the BBB and penetration of harmful substances into the brain tissue [17]. These agents activate microglia and astrocytes to produce pro-inflammatory cytokines, which cause neuroinflammation. While neuroinflammation is a normal physiological process that protects the brain environment from infection, toxic agents, and misfolding proteins, chronic cerebral inflammation exerts detrimental consequences in the CNS [184]. Microglia are identified by several surface receptors (CD11b, CD45, CX3CR1, CD16, CD40, CD80, CD68, CD115, and others) and intracellular proteins (IBA1, Pu.1, HexB, vimentin, and Sall1) in the CNS [185–192]. Functionally, there are two distinct states of microglia. The resting or ramified microglia represent round cell bodies and vigorous branching processes, which constitute a large part of cerebral microglia in physiological conditions. Under pathological conditions (PAMPs, DAMPs, and toxic substances in the brain), amoeboid form or activated microglia are the dominant state. Microglia in this form are less branched and have round cell bodies with thick processes that make it easier to move toward injury sites [193–196]. Just like liver KCs, microglia can be classified phenotypically into two types: M1 (pro-inflammatory phenotype) and M2 (anti-inflammatory). The M1 microglia ($CD14^+$, $CD16^+$, $CD40^+$, $CD32^+$, $CD86^{+,}$ and $MHCII^+$) often triggered by pro-inflammatory factors such as TNFα, IFNγ, and LPS, which cause the production of pro-inflammatory mediators. M2 microglia ($CD163^+$ and $CD206^+$) in response to IL-13, TGFβ, IL-4, and IL-10 secrete anti-inflammatory mediators and neurotropic factors, including IL-13, CCL22, CCL17, IL-10, brain-derived neurotrophic factor (BDNF), CSF-1, glial cell-derived neurotrophic factor (GDNF), nerve growth factor (NGF), and TGFβ [197, 198].

Following cirrhosis, hyperammonemia, and systemic inflammation may interrupt the function of tight junction proteins and impair the integrity of the BBB (**Table 3**) [229–231]. Hyperammonemia, systemic inflammation, and enhanced BBB permeability were found in mice with BDL as a model for chronic liver disease-induced HE [8]. Similar findings were also revealed in CCL4-induced cirrhosis in rats [232]. Likewise, disruption of the BBB and decreased mRNA and protein expression of tight junction proteins (i.e. claudin-5, occludin, and ZO-1) were demonstrated in a BDL-rat model of HE [205]. Furthermore, systemic inflammation, hyperammonemia, and a decrease in the expression of thigh junction proteins were revealed in mice after the injection of

Study	Findings (Brain tissue)	References
Rodrigo et al. (2010)	⇧MHCII, ⇧iNOS, ⇧IL-1β, ⇧PGE2, ⇧ammonia (BDL rats)	[199]
Claeys et al. (2022)	⇧Astrocyte reactivity (⇧GFAP), ⇧microglial activation, ⇧BBB permeabilization (BDL mice)	[8]
Tamnanloo et al. (2023)	⇧Cleaved caspase-3, ⇧IL-1β, ⇧TNFα, ⇧Bax/Bcl2 ratio, ⇧oxidative stress, ⇩total antioxidant capacity (BDL rats)	[200]
Bosoi et al. (2012)	⇧Brain water content, ⇧ammonia in cerebrospinal fluid (CSF) (BDL rats)	[201]
Magen et al. (2009)	⇧TNFR1 mRNA, ⇩BDNF mRNA, ⇩A2A adenosine receptor (BDL mice)	[202]
André Clément et al. (2020)	⇩NeuN, ⇧cleaved caspase-3, ⇧neuronal apoptosis	[203]
Stojanović et al. (2023)	⇩Catalase, ⇩superoxide dismutase activities, ⇩glutathione, ⇩peroxidase activity, ⇧lipid peroxidation, ⇧iNOS (CCL4 rats)	[204]
Dhanda et al. (2018)	⇧BBB permeabilization, ⇧brain water content, ⇧aquaporin-4 mRNA and protein, ⇧MMP-9 mRNA and protein, ⇩mRNA and protein occludin, ⇩mRNA and protein claudin-5, ⇩mRNA and protein ZO-1 (BDL rats)	[205]
Yang et al. (2015)	⇩BrdU (neurogenesis), ⇩NeuN (post-mitotic neurons) ⇩GFAP (astrocytes) (CCL4 rats)	[206]
Golshani et al. (2019)	⇧degenerative cerebellar Purkinje neurons, ⇧degenerative hippocampal pyramidal neurons, ⇧GFAP, ⇧CD11+ (BDL rats)	[207]
Jung Hsu et al. (2021)	⇧Iba1, ⇧IL-1β, ⇧IFNγ, ⇧TNFα, ⇧IGF-1, ⇧VEGFD (BDL rats)	[208]
Chen et al. (2014)	⇧Microglia activation, ⇧GFAP, ⇩dendritic spine density (BDL rats)	[209]
Chen et al. 2012	⇧NADPH-dependent superoxide anion, ⇧BBB disruption (BDL rats)	[210]
Pierzchala et al. (2022)	⇧8-Oxo-2′-deoxyguanosine, ⇧IL-6, ⇧glutathione peroxidase 1, ⇧superoxide dismutase, ⇧MnSOD (BDL rats)	[211]
Ahmadi et al. (2020)	⇧Jnk3 mRNA, ⇧JNK3 protein (BDL rats)	[212]
Y Avraham et al. (2010)	⇧TNFR1 mRNA, ⇩BDNF mRNA, ⇩5-HT1A receptor (BDL mice)	[213]
M.V. Gee et al. (2023)	⇩Astrocyte covering BBB, ⇧neuronal senescence, ⇩neuronal connectivity (BDL mice)	[214]
Shabani et al. (2019)	⇧Neuronal loss, ⇧neuronal apoptosis (BDL rats)	[215]
Balasubramaniyan et al. (2012)	⇧Brain water content, ⇧TNFα, ⇧NOX-1 protein, (BDL rats)	[216]
Dhanda et al. (2018)	⇧IL-6 mRNA and protein, ⇧TNFα mRNA and protein, ⇧MCP-1 mRNA and protein, ⇩Iba1 expression, ⇩GFAP expression, ⇩BDNF (BDL rats)	[156]
Wright et al. (2010)	⇧Ammonia, ⇧TNFα, ⇧IL-6, ⇧brain water content, ⇧iNOS, ⇧IL-1β, ⇧GFAP, ⇧TGFβ mRNA (BDL rats)	[217]
Faropoulos et al. (2010)	⇧Superoxide radical, ⇩occludin (BDL rats)	[218]
Boer et al. (2009)	⇩Activity of mitochondrial complexes I, II and IV (CCL4 rats)	[219]

Study	Findings (Brain tissue)	References
Liu et al. (2020)	⇧IL1β mRNA, ⇧MCP-1 mRNA, ⇧IBA1 mRNA, ⇧GFAP mRNA, ⇧NeuN/Fox3 (CCL4 mice)	[14]
Khan et al. (2019)	⇧IL-1β, ⇧IL-6, ⇧TNFα, ⇩glutathione, ⇩catalase, ⇧malondialdehyde, ⇧nitrite, ⇩GFAP, ⇩BDNF, ⇩VEGF, ⇧apoptosis (CCL4 mice)	[220]
Machado et al. (2015)	⇧TNFα, ⇧IL-1β, ⇧IL-18, IL-6 (unchanged), IL-10 (unchanged) (CCL4 rats)	[221]
Hadjihambi et al. (2018)	⇩AQP4, ⇩glymphatic clearance (BDL rats)	[222]
Jung Hsu et al. (2021)	⇧NF-κβ mRNA, ⇧Iba1mRNA, ⇧TNFα mRNA (Cirrhosis patients with HE)	[208]
Irina et al. (2021)	⇧Iba1, cytokines unchanged (postmortem; cirrhosis patients with HE)	[223]
Boris et al. (2013)	Change in the expression patterns of genes related to oxidative stress, microglia activation, inflammatory signaling, cell proliferation, and apoptosis (postmortem; cirrhosis patients with HE)	[224]
Grover et al. (2011)	⇧PK11195 binding, a ligand for activated microglia (patients with chronic hepatitis C)	[225]
Balzano et al. (2018)	⇧Purkinje cell loss, ⇧neuronal loss in granular layer, ⇧microglial activation, ⇧reactive astrocytes, ⇧degeneration of Bergmann glia, ⇧lymphocytes infiltration (postmortem; cirrhosis patients with HE)	[226]
Cagnin et al. (2006)	⇧PK11195 binding, a ligand for activated glial cells (patients with cirrhosis)	[227]
Butterworth et al. (1988)	⇧Dysfunctional astrocytes (astrogliosis) (postmortem; cirrhosis patients with HE)	[228]

Table 3.
Main cerebral changes following cirrhosis and HE.

CCL4 [233, 234]. Quinn et al. demonstrated elevated circulating bile acids increase the permeability of the BBB through a detrimental impact on tight junction proteins in BDL rats [235]. Elevated circulatory ammonia (unprotonated form; NH_3) can passively diffuse into the brain parenchyma. Moreover, several transporting systems (i.e., aquaporins, Na^+/H^+ exchangers, Na^+/K^+-ATPase, and potassium channels) mediated ammonia transportation (ionic form; NH_4^+) across the BBB [236–240]. Disrupted integrity of the BBB and tight junction proteins leads to exposure of brain tissue to high levels of harmful circulatory substances, including LPS, pro-inflammatory cytokines, chemokines, ammonia, bacterial DNA, DAMPs, and bile acids (**Figure 3**). In addition to impaired BBB, several reported pathways were identified for the entry of systemic cytokines into the brain parenchyma: peripheral vagus nerve, circumventricular organs, recruitment of activated circulatory immune cells, and activated capillary endothelial cells that produce pro-inflammatory cytokines in the brain parenchyma [241–244]. Elevated levels of DAMPs (i.e., HMGB1, ATP, bacterial DNA segments, and apoptotic bodies), pro-inflammatory cytokines, ammonia, LPS, bacterial metabolites, and their components in the brain parenchyma trigger microglia through activation of their TLR2, TLR4, TLR9, NOD2, RAGE, and purinergic receptors, resulting in change in their phenotypes from resting-branched to active-amoeboid state (**Figure 3**). The activated microglia produce and secrete pro-inflammatory mediators, including IL-1β, TNFα, IL-6, IL-12, CCL2, iNOS, IL-23,

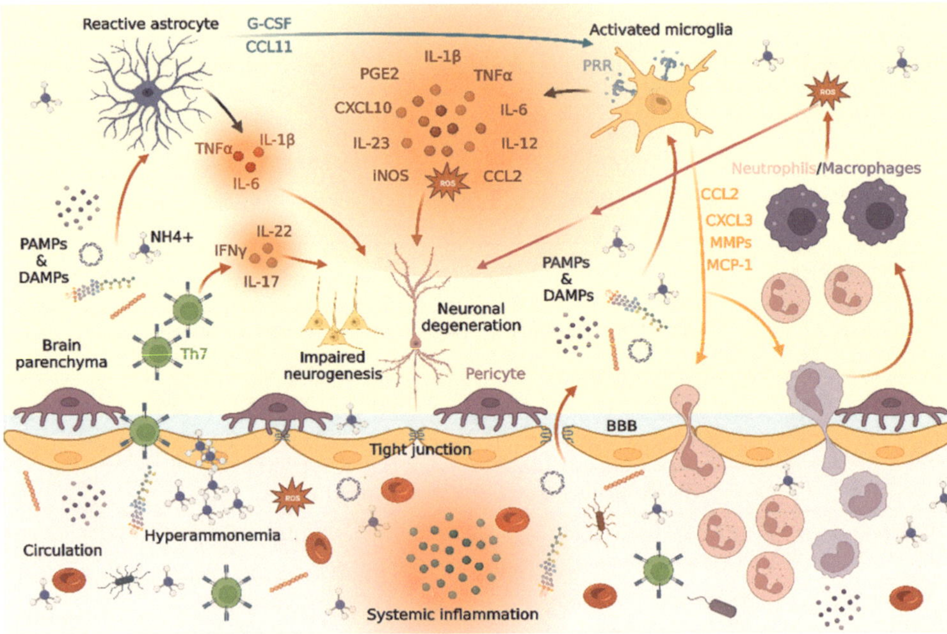

Figure 3.
Hyperammonemia, systemic inflammation, and gut-derived compounds disrupt the integrity of the blood-brain barrier and induce neuroinflammation in cirrhosis, highlighting the role of brain-activated microglia. BBB, blood-brain barrier; DAMPs, damage-associated molecular pattern molecules; CCL2, C-C motif chemokine ligand 2; CCL11, C-C motif chemokine ligand 11; CXCL3, C-X-C motif chemokine ligand 3; CXCL10, C-X-C motif chemokine ligand 10; G-CSF, granulocyte colony-stimulating factor; iNOS, inducible nitric oxide synthases; IFNγ, interferon gamma; IL-1β, Interleukin-1 beta; IL-6, Interleukin-6; IL-12, Interleukin-12; IL-17, Interleukin-17; IL-22, Interleukin-22; IL-23, Interleukin-23; MCP-1, monocyte chemoattractant protein-1; MMPs, matrix metalloproteinases; NH_4^+, ammonia; PAMPs, pathogen-associated molecular patterns; PGE2, prostaglandin E_2; PRR, pattern recognition receptors; ROS, reactive oxygen species; TNFα, tumor necrosis factor alpha. Created with BioRender.com.

CXCL10, and PGE2, which progress the induction of oxidative stress and neuroinflammation (**Figure 3**). Chronic neuroinflammation in response to elevated cerebral levels of PAMPS, DAMPs, and ammonia induces neuronal loss and impairs neurogenesis, resulting in neurodegeneration and encephalopathy [199, 223, 224, 245–252]. Interestingly, postmortem brain examinations of cirrhotic individuals with HE showed up-regulation of genes related to oxidative stress, inflammatory pathways, and microglial activation [224]. Hyperammonemia in BDL rats triggered microglial activation, increased cerebral levels of iNOS, PGE2, and IL-1β, and progressed motor dysfunction, as well as impaired cognitive functions [199]. Microglia activation and increased population of $CD11^+$ cells, as well as an increase in the number of degenerative neurons demonstrated in the hippocampus and cerebellum of BDL rats [207]. Moreover, increased expression of microglia marker Iba1 and cerebral ammonia were seen in the prefrontal cortex of BDL mice [8]. Increased lipid peroxidation, decreased total antioxidant capacity, infiltrated leukocytes, and injured neuronal cells were observed in the brain tissues of CCL4-induced cirrhosis rats [253]. In addition, mouse models of liver fibrosis by CCL4 showed increased mRNA expression of IL-1β, TGF-β1, and matrix metalloproteinase-9 (MMP9) in the brain parenchyma [234]. Likewise, mRNA and protein levels of MMP9 and VCAM-1 were up-regulated in different brain regions of BDL rats [205]. Activated microglia also stimulate the recruitment of circulatory monocytes and neutrophils into brain tissue through their secretory chemoattractant agents, CCL2, MCP-1, CXCL3, and MMPs (**Figure 3**) [254–256]. In a mouse model of chronic liver failure due to bile duct resection, activated brain microglia with a mechanism dependent on TNFα-TNF receptor 1 (TNFR1)-produced CCL2 and MCP-1 stimulate monocyte chemotaxis into the brain [256]. Cerebral astrocytes (glial fibrillary acidic protein; GFAP) are directly exposed to ammonia and circulatory PAMPs and DAMPs. These agents changed the astrocyte state from resting to a reactive form that produced pro-inflammatory mediators and induced oxidative stress. Afterward, reactive astrocytes activate microglia through secretion of G-CSF and CCL11 [257–260]. Moreover, activated microglia, *via* production of GM-CSF, TNFα, and IL-1β trigger astrocytes to produce pro-inflammatory cytokines that exacerbate neuroinflammation [231]. Hyperammonemic cerebral conditions induce astrocyte swelling and brain edema through mislocalization of aquaporin four water channels, inflammation, TLR4 activation, mitochondrial dysfunction, glutamine accumulation, and induction of oxidative stress [7, 257, 261]. Although cerebral edema often progresses in acute forms of HE, patients with cirrhosis were found to have minimal levels of brain edema using ^{1}H-magnetic resonance (MR) spectroscopy [262]. Systemic inflammation, hyperammonemia, an abnormal phenotype of astrocytes (thin chromatin and enlarged nuclei), and increased brain water content (an indicator of cerebral edema) were demonstrated in BDL rats [263]. Moreover, in other experimental models of cirrhosis-induced HE, astrogliosis, gliopathy, neuroinflammation, and raise in brain water content were observed [8, 207, 233, 234, 248, 264].

5. Conclusion

While the pathophysiology of cirrhosis-induced HE remains to be elucidated, the progression of cirrhosis and HE is associated with innate immune disturbances at different levels of the gut-liver-brain axis. In cirrhosis, gut dysbiosis and bacterial overgrowth cause intestinal barrier disruption, leading to bacterial translocation and activation of intestinal Mϕ and DCs that initiate tissue inflammation. Bacterial metabolites, ammonia, and gut-derived inflammatory cytokines reach the hepatic sinusoids and activate HSCs and KCs, resulting in the production of liver inflammation and the induction of oxidative stress and exacerbate systemic inflammation. Also, injured hepatocytes cannot detoxify ammonia, resulting in hyperammonemia. Systemic inflammation, hyperammonemia, and endotoxemia induce the BBB injury and allow brain tissue to be exposed to all circulatory neurotoxic substances. These agents stimulate brain microglia to produce pro-inflammatory cytokines and induce oxidative stress in the CNS. Neuroinflammation and oxidative stress decrease neurogenesis and induce neuronal degeneration, resulting in neurological and psychological manifestations seen in HE. Due to the implication of Mϕ, immune cells and inflammation in different levels of gut-liver-brain axis, they can be potent therapeutic targets for future experimental and clinical research to find an all-encompassing treatment option that targets restoration of the immune system in multiple organs following cirrhosis and HE.

Conflict of interest

The authors declare no conflict of interest.

Author details

Ali Sepehrinezhad[1,2]* and Ali Shahbazi[1,3]*

1 Department of Neuroscience, Faculty of Advanced Technologies in Medicine, Iran University of Medical Sciences, Tehran, Iran

2 Neuroscience Research Center, Mashhad University of Medical Sciences, Mashhad, Iran

3 Cellular and Molecular Research Center, Iran University of Medical Sciences, Tehran, Iran

*Address all correspondence to: sepehrinezhad.a@iums.ac.ir and shahbazi.a@iums.ac.ir

References

[1] Rose CF, Amodio P, Bajaj JS, et al. Hepatic encephalopathy: Novel insights into classification, pathophysiology and therapy. Journal of Hepatology. 2020;**73**: 1526-1547. DOI: 10.1016/j.jhep.2020.07.013

[2] Ochoa-Sanchez R, Rose CF. Pathogenesis of hepatic encephalopathy in chronic liver disease. Journal of Clinical and Experimental Hepatology. 2018;**8**:262-271. DOI: 10.1016/j.jceh.2018.08.001

[3] Jalan R, Rose CF. Heretical thoughts into hepatic encephalopathy. Journal of Hepatology. 2022;**77**:539-548. DOI: 10.1016/j.jhep.2022.03.014

[4] Montagnese S, Russo FP, Amodio P, et al. Hepatic encephalopathy 2018: A clinical practice guideline by the Italian Association for the Study of the liver (AISF). Digestive and Liver Disease. 2019;**51**:190-205. DOI: 10.1016/j.dld.2018.11.035

[5] Weissenborn K. Hepatic encephalopathy: Definition, clinical grading and diagnostic principles. Drugs. 2019;**79**:5-9. DOI: 10.1007/s40265-018-1018-z

[6] Kroupina K, Bémeur C, Rose CF. Amino acids, ammonia, and hepatic encephalopathy. Analytical Biochemistry. 2022;**649**:114696

[7] Sepehrinezhad A, Zarifkar A, Namvar G, et al. Astrocyte swelling in hepatic encephalopathy: Molecular perspective of cytotoxic edema. Metabolic Brain Disease. 2020;**35**: 559-578. DOI: 10.1007/s11011-020-00549-8

[8] Claeys W, Van Hoecke L, Geerts A, et al. A mouse model of hepatic encephalopathy: Bile duct ligation induces brain ammonia overload, glial cell activation and neuroinflammation. Scientific Reports. 2022;**12**:17558. DOI: 10.1038/s41598-022-22423-6

[9] Shawcross D, Jalan R. The pathophysiologic basis of hepatic encephalopathy: Central role for ammonia and inflammation. Cellular and Molecular Life Sciences CMLS. 2005;**62**:2295-2304. DOI: 10.1007/s00018-005-5089-0

[10] Shawcross DL, Wright G, Olde Damink SWM, et al. Role of ammonia and inflammation in minimal hepatic encephalopathy. Metabolic Brain Disease. 2007;**22**:125-138. DOI: 10.1007/s11011-006-9042-1

[11] Aldridge DR, Tranah EJ, Shawcross DL. Pathogenesis of hepatic encephalopathy: Role of ammonia and systemic inflammation. Journal of Clinical and Experimental Hepatology. 2015;**5**:S7-S20. DOI: 10.1016/j.jceh.2014.06.004

[12] Tranah TH, Vijay GK, Ryan JM, et al. Systemic inflammation and ammonia in hepatic encephalopathy. Metabolic Brain Disease. 2013;**28**:1-5. DOI: 10.1007/s11011-012-9370-2

[13] Laguna, de la Vera A-L, Welsch C, Pfeilschifter W, et al. Chapter 8 - gut–liver–brain axis in chronic liver disease with a focus on hepatic encephalopathy. In: Stasi C, editor. The Complex Interplay between Gut-Brain, Gut-Liver, and Liver-Brain Axes. London, United Kingdom: Academic Press; 2021. pp. 159-185

[14] Liu R, Kang JD, Sartor RB, et al. Neuroinflammation in murine cirrhosis

is dependent on the gut microbiome and is attenuated by fecal transplant. Hepatology. 2020;**71**:611-626

[15] Kang DJ, Betrapally NS, Ghosh SA, et al. Gut microbiota drive the development of neuroinflammatory response in cirrhosis in mice. Hepatology. 2016;**64**:1232-1248

[16] Jain L, Sharma BC, Srivastava S, et al. Serum endotoxin, inflammatory mediators, and magnetic resonance spectroscopy before and after treatment in patients with minimal hepatic encephalopathy. Journal of Gastroenterology and Hepatology. 2013; **28**:1187-1193

[17] Shahbazi A, Sepehrinezhad A, Vahdani E, et al. Gut dysbiosis and blood-brain barrier alteration in hepatic encephalopathy: From gut to brain. Biomedicine. 2023;**11**:1272

[18] Wu H, Zhang Y, Yu J, et al. Gut-liver-brain axis: A complex network influences human health and diseases. Frontiers in Neuroscience. 2023;**17**: 1241069

[19] Nguyen HH, Swain MG. Avenues within the gut-liver-brain axis linking chronic liver disease and symptoms. Frontiers in Neuroscience. 2023;**17**:1171253

[20] Beldowska A, Barszcz M, Dunislawska A. State of the art in research on the gut-liver and gut-brain axis in poultry. Journal of Animal Science and Biotechnology. 2023;**14**:37

[21] Ding JH, Jin Z, Yang XX, et al. Role of gut microbiota via the gut-liver-brain axis in digestive diseases. World Journal of Gastroenterology. 2020;**26**:6141-6162. DOI: 10.3748/wjg.v26.i40.6141

[22] Krakovski MA, Arora N, Jain S, et al. Diet-microbiome-gut-brain nexus in acute and chronic brain injury. Frontiers in Neuroscience. 2022;**16**:1002266. DOI: 10.3389/fnins.2022.1002266

[23] Sepehrinezhad A, Shahbazi A, Joghataei MT, et al. Inhibition of autotaxin alleviates pathological features of hepatic encephalopathy at the level of gut–liver–brain axis: An experimental and bioinformatic study. Cell Death & Disease. 2023;**14**:490

[24] Luo M, Xin R-J, Hu F-R, et al. Role of gut microbiota in the pathogenesis and therapeutics of minimal hepatic encephalopathy via the gut-liver-brain axis. World Journal of Gastroenterology. 2023;**29**:144

[25] Ahluwalia V, Betrapally NS, Hylemon PB, et al. Impaired gut-liver-brain axis in patients with cirrhosis. Scientific Reports. 2016;**6**:26800. DOI: 10.1038/srep26800

[26] Fogg DK, Sibon C, Miled C, et al. A clonogenic bone marrow progenitor specific for macrophages and dendritic cells. Science. 2006;**311**:83-87

[27] van Furth R, Cohn ZA. The origin and kinetics of mononuclear phagocytes. The Journal of Experimental Medicine. 1968;**128**:415-435

[28] Cerovic V, Bain CC, Mowat AM, et al. Intestinal macrophages and dendritic cells: what's the difference? Trends in Immunology. 2014;**35**:270-277

[29] Zhang F, Wang H, Wang X, et al. TGF-β induces M2-like macrophage polarization via SNAIL-mediated suppression of a pro-inflammatory phenotype. Oncotarget. 2016;**7**: 52294-52306. DOI: 10.18632/oncotarget.10561

[30] Gong D, Shi W, Yi S-J, et al. TGFβ signaling plays a critical role in

promoting alternative macrophage activation. BMC Immunology. 2012;**13**: 31. DOI: 10.1186/1471-2172-13-31

[31] Boulakirba S, Pfeifer A, Mhaidly R, et al. IL-34 and CSF-1 display an equivalent macrophage differentiation ability but a different polarization potential. Scientific Reports. 2018;**8**:256. DOI: 10.1038/s41598-017-18433-4

[32] Schridde A, Bain CC, Mayer JU, et al. Tissue-specific differentiation of colonic macrophages requires TGFβ receptor-mediated signaling. Mucosal Immunology. 2017;**10**:1387-1399. DOI: 10.1038/mi.2016.142

[33] Kumawat AK, Yu C, Mann EA, et al. Expression and characterization of αvβ5 integrin on intestinal macrophages. European Journal of Immunology. 2018; **48**:1181-1187

[34] Henson PM. Cell removal: efferocytosis. Annual Review of Cell and Developmental Biology. 2017;**33**:127-144

[35] Cosin-Roger J, Ortiz-Masià MD, Barrachina MD. Macrophages as an emerging source of Wnt ligands: Relevance in mucosal integrity. Frontiers in Immunology. 2019;**10**:2297. DOI: 10.3389/fimmu.2019.02297

[36] Chikina AS, Nadalin F, Maurin M, et al. Macrophages maintain epithelium integrity by limiting fungal product absorption. Cell. 2020;**183**(411–428): e416

[37] D'Angelo F, Bernasconi E, Schäfer M, et al. Macrophages promote epithelial repair through hepatocyte growth factor secretion. Clinical and Experimental Immunology. 2013;**174**: 60-72. DOI: 10.1111/cei.12157

[38] Na YR, Jung D, Stakenborg M, et al. Prostaglandin E(2) receptor PTGER4-expressing macrophages promote intestinal epithelial barrier regeneration upon inflammation. Gut. 2021;**70**: 2249-2260. DOI: 10.1136/gutjnl-2020-322146

[39] Viola MF, Boeckxstaens G. Niche-specific functional heterogeneity of intestinal resident macrophages. Gut. 2021;**70**:1383-1395

[40] Muller PA, Koscsó B, Rajani GM, et al. Crosstalk between muscularis macrophages and enteric neurons regulates gastrointestinal motility. Cell. 2014;**158**:300-313. DOI: 10.1016/j.cell.2014.04.050

[41] Luo J, Qian A, Oetjen LK, et al. TRPV4 channel signaling in macrophages promotes gastrointestinal motility via direct effects on smooth muscle cells. Immunity. 2018;**49**: 107-119.e104. DOI: 10.1016/j.immuni.2018.04.021

[42] Avetisyan M, Rood JE, Huerta Lopez S, et al. Muscularis macrophage development in the absence of an enteric nervous system. Proceedings of the National Academy of Sciences. 2018;**115**: 4696-4701. DOI: 10.1073/pnas.1802490115

[43] Bajaj JS, Betrapally NS, Hylemon PB, et al. Salivary microbiota reflects changes in gut microbiota in cirrhosis with hepatic encephalopathy. Hepatology. 2015;**62**:1260-1271. DOI: 10.1002/hep.27819

[44] Zhang Z, Zhai H, Geng J, et al. Large-scale survey of gut microbiota associated with MHE via 16S rRNA-based pyrosequencing. American College of Gastroenterology. 2013;**108**:1601-1611

[45] Wang WW, Zhang Y, Huang XB, et al. Fecal microbiota transplantation prevents hepatic encephalopathy in rats

with carbon tetrachloride-induced acute hepatic dysfunction. World Journal of Gastroenterology. 2017;**23**:6983-6994. DOI: 10.3748/wjg.v23.i38.6983

[46] Wang L, Cui H, Li Y, et al. Kang-Xian pills inhibit inflammatory response and decrease gut permeability to treat carbon tetrachloride-induced chronic hepatic injury through modulating gut microbiota. Evidence-based Complementary and Alternative Medicine. 2020;**2020**:8890182. DOI: 10.1155/2020/8890182

[47] Zhou K, Jiang M, Liu Y, et al. Effect of bile pigments on the compromised gut barrier function in a rat model of bile duct ligation. PLoS One. 2014;**9**:e98905. DOI: 10.1371/journal.pone.0098905

[48] Wang C, Ma C, Fu K, et al. Phillygenin attenuates carbon tetrachloride-induced liver fibrosis via modulating inflammation and gut microbiota. Frontiers in Pharmacology. 2021;**12**. DOI: 10.3389/fphar.2021.756924

[49] Luyer MDP, Buurman WA, Hadfoune M, et al. High-fat enteral nutrition reduces endotoxin, tumor necrosis factor-alpha and gut permeability in bile duct-ligated rats subjected to hemorrhagic shock. Journal of Hepatology. 2004;**41**:377-383. DOI: 10.1016/j.jhep.2004.04.026

[50] Palma P, Mihaljevic N, Hasenberg T, et al. Intestinal barrier dysfunction in developing liver cirrhosis: An *in vivo* analysis of bacterial translocation. Hepatology Research. 2007;**37**:6-12. DOI: 10.1111/j.1872-034X.2007.00004.x

[51] Lei W, Zhao C, Sun J, et al. Electroacupuncture ameliorates intestinal barrier destruction in mice with bile duct ligation–induced liver injury by activating the cholinergic anti-inflammatory pathway. Neuromodulation. 2022;**25**:1122-1133. DOI: 10.1016/j.neurom.2022.02.001

[52] Fu K, Ma C, Wang C, et al. Forsythiaside A alleviated carbon tetrachloride-induced liver fibrosis by modulating gut microbiota composition to increase short-chain fatty acids and restoring bile acids metabolism disorder. Biomedicine & Pharmacotherapy. 2022; **151**:113185. DOI: 10.1016/j.biopha.2022.113185

[53] Sánchez E, Nieto JC, Boullosa A, et al. VSL#3 probiotic treatment decreases bacterial translocation in rats with carbon tetrachloride-induced cirrhosis. Liver International. 2015;**35**: 735-745. DOI: 10.1111/liv.12566

[54] Cabrera-Rubio R, Patterson AM, Cotter PD, et al. Cholestasis induced by bile duct ligation promotes changes in the intestinal microbiome in mice. Scientific Reports. 2019;**9**:12324. DOI: 10.1038/s41598-019-48784-z

[55] Zhao T, Zhu Y, Yao L, et al. IGF-1 alleviates CCL4-induced hepatic cirrhosis and dysfunction of intestinal barrier through inhibition TLR4/NF-κB signaling mediated by down-regulation HMGB1. Annals of Hepatology. 2021;**26**: 100560. DOI: 10.1016/j.aohep.2021.100560

[56] Safari F, Sharifi M, Talebi A, et al. Alleviation of cholestatic liver injury and intestinal permeability by lubiprostone treatment in bile duct ligated rats: Role of intestinal FXR and tight junction proteins claudin-1, claudin-2, and occludin. Naunyn-Schmiedeberg's Archives of Pharmacology. 2023;**396**: 2009-2022. DOI: 10.1007/s00210-023-02455-z

[57] Assimakopoulos SF, Vagianos CE, Patsoukis N, et al. Evidence for intestinal oxidative stress in obstructive jaundice-

induced gut barrier dysfunction in rats. Acta Physiologica Scandinavica. 2004; **180**:177-185. DOI: 10.1046/j.0001-6772.2003.01229.x

[58] Chen Y, Qin N, Guo J, et al. Functional gene arrays-based analysis of fecal microbiomes in patients with liver cirrhosis. BMC Genomics. 2014;**15**:753. DOI: 10.1186/1471-2164-15-753

[59] Assimakopoulos SF, Tsamandas AC, Tsiaoussis GI, et al. Intestinal mucosal proliferation, apoptosis and oxidative stress in patients with liver cirrhosis. Annals of Hepatology. 2015;**12**:301-307

[60] Chen Y, Yang F, Lu H, et al. Characterization of fecal microbial communities in patients with liver cirrhosis. Hepatology. 2011;**54**:562-572. DOI: 10.1002/hep.24423

[61] Du Plessis J, Vanheel H, Janssen CEI, et al. Activated intestinal macrophages in patients with cirrhosis release NO and IL-6 that may disrupt intestinal barrier function. Journal of Hepatology. 2013;**58**: 1125-1132. DOI: 10.1016/j.jhep.2013.01.038

[62] Pascual S, Such J, Esteban A, et al. Intestinal permeability is increased in patients with advanced cirrhosis. Hepato-Gastroenterology. 2003;**50**: 1482-1486

[63] Yang B, Sun T, Chen Y, et al. The role of gut microbiota in mice with bile duct ligation-evoked cholestatic liver disease-related cognitive dysfunction. Frontiers in Microbiology. 2022;**13**: 909461

[64] Đurašević S, Pejić S, Grigorov I, et al. Effects of C60 fullerene on thioacetamide-induced rat liver toxicity and gut microbiome changes. Antioxidants. 2021;**10**:911

[65] De Minicis S, Rychlicki C, Agostinelli L, et al. Dysbiosis contributes to fibrogenesis in the course of chronic liver injury in mice. Hepatology. 2014; **59**:1738-1749

[66] Li Y, Lv L, Ye J, et al. Bifidobacterium adolescentis CGMCC 15058 alleviates liver injury, enhances the intestinal barrier and modifies the gut microbiota in D-galactosamine-treated rats. Applied Microbiology and Biotechnology. 2019;**103**:375-393

[67] Muñoz L, Borrero MJ, Úbeda M, et al. Intestinal immune dysregulation driven by dysbiosis promotes barrier disruption and bacterial translocation in rats with cirrhosis. Hepatology. 2019;**70**: 925-938. DOI: 10.1002/hep.30349

[68] Qin N, Yang F, Li A, et al. Alterations of the human gut microbiome in liver cirrhosis. Nature. 2014;**513**:59-64. DOI: 10.1038/nature13568

[69] Úbeda M, Lario M, Muñoz L, et al. Obeticholic acid reduces bacterial translocation and inhibits intestinal inflammation in cirrhotic rats. Journal of Hepatology. 2016;**64**:1049-1057

[70] Such J, Guardiola JV, de Juan J, et al. Ultrastructural characteristics of distal duodenum mucosa in patients with cirrhosis. European Journal of Gastroenterology & Hepatology. 2002; **14**:371-376

[71] Ramachandran A, Prabhu R, Thomas S, et al. Intestinal mucosal alterations in experimental cirrhosis in the rat: Role of oxygen free radicals. Hepatology. 2002;**35**:622-629

[72] Reiberger T, Ferlitsch A, Payer BA, et al. Non-selective betablocker therapy decreases intestinal permeability and serum levels of LBP and IL-6 in patients

with cirrhosis. Journal of Hepatology. 2013;**58**:911-921

[73] Kaliannan K. Compromise of α-defensin function in liver cirrhosis facilitates the toxic relationship between gut permeability and endotoxemia. Digestive Diseases and Sciences. 2018; **63**:2492-2494. DOI: 10.1007/s10620-018-5197-y

[74] Wiest R, Lawson M, Geuking M. Pathological bacterial translocation in liver cirrhosis. Journal of Hepatology. 2014;**60**:197-209. DOI: 10.1016/j.jhep.2013.07.044

[75] Yan AW, Fouts DE, Brandl J, et al. Enteric dysbiosis associated with a mouse model of alcoholic liver disease. Hepatology. 2011;**53**:96-105

[76] Tsiaoussis GI, Assimakopoulos SF, Tsamandas AC, et al. Intestinal barrier dysfunction in cirrhosis: Current concepts in pathophysiology and clinical implications. World Journal of Hepatology. 2015;7:2058-2068. DOI: 10.4254/wjh.v7.i17.2058

[77] Chen S, Li X, Li M, et al. Mucosal expression of defensin-5, soluble phospholipase A2 and lysozyme in the intestine in a rat model of acute liver failure and its relationship to intestinal bacterial translocation. Gastroenterología y Hepatología. 2020; **43**:293-300. DOI: 10.1016/j.gastrohep.2020.01.004

[78] Teltschik Z, Wiest R, Beisner J, et al. Intestinal bacterial translocation in rats with cirrhosis is related to compromised paneth cell antimicrobial host defense. Hepatology. 2012;**55**:1154-1163. DOI: 10.1002/hep.24789

[79] Irvine KM, Ratnasekera I, Powell EE, et al. Causes and consequences of innate immune dysfunction in cirrhosis. Frontiers in Immunology. 2019;**10**:293. DOI: 10.3389/fimmu.2019.00293

[80] Wiest R, Garcia-Tsao G. Bacterial translocation (BT) in cirrhosis. Hepatology. 2005;**41**:422-433. DOI: 10.1002/hep.20632

[81] Riva A, Gray EH, Azarian S, et al. Faecal cytokine profiling as a marker of intestinal inflammation in acutely decompensated cirrhosis. JHEP Reports. 2020;**2**:100151. DOI: 10.1016/j.jhepr.2020.100151

[82] Assimakopoulos SF, Tsamandas AC, Tsiaoussis GI, et al. Altered intestinal tight junctions' expression in patients with liver cirrhosis: A pathogenetic mechanism of intestinal hyperpermeability. European Journal of Clinical Investigation. 2012;**42**: 439-446. DOI: 10.1111/j.1365-2362.2011.02609.x

[83] Muñoz L, Albillos A, Nieto M, et al. Mesenteric Th1 polarization and monocyte TNF-α production: First steps to systemic inflammation in rats with cirrhosis. Hepatology. 2005;**42**:411-419

[84] Munoz L, Jose Borrero M, Ubeda M, et al. Interaction between intestinal dendritic cells and bacteria translocated from the gut in rats with cirrhosis. Hepatology. 2012;**56**:1861-1869

[85] Úbeda M, Munoz L, Borrero MJ, et al. Critical role of the liver in the induction of systemic inflammation in rats with preascitic cirrhosis. Hepatology. 2010;**52**:2086-2095

[86] Munoz L, Borrero M-J, Ubeda M, et al. Commensal gut flora drives the expansion of proinflammatory T cells in the small intestinal mucosa in rats with CCl4 cirrhosis. In: Hepatology. NJ, USA: Wiley-Blackwell; 2013. p. 985A

[87] Albillos A, Lario M, Álvarez-Mon M. Cirrhosis-associated immune dysfunction: Distinctive features and clinical relevance. Journal of Hepatology. 2014;**61**:1385-1396. DOI: 10.1016/j.jhep.2014.08.010

[88] Iwasaki A, Medzhitov R. Toll-like receptor control of the adaptive immune responses. Nature Immunology. 2004;**5**: 987-995

[89] McClure R, Massari P. TLR-dependent human mucosal epithelial cell responses to microbial pathogens. Frontiers in Immunology. 2014;**5**:386

[90] Kawai T, Akira S. The role of pattern-recognition receptors in innate immunity: Update on toll-like receptors. Nature Immunology. 2010;**11**:373-384

[91] Kawasaki T, Kawai T. Toll-like receptor signaling pathways. Frontiers in Immunology. 2014;**5**:461

[92] Fitzgerald KA, Kagan JC. Toll-like receptors and the control of immunity. Cell. 2020;**180**:1044-1066

[93] Schnare M, Barton GM, Holt AC, et al. Toll-like receptors control activation of adaptive immune responses. Nature Immunology. 2001;**2**: 947-950

[94] Lan YT, Wang ZL, Tian P, et al. Treg/Th17 imbalance and its clinical significance in patients with hepatitis B-associated liver cirrhosis. Diagnostic Pathology. 2019;**14**:114. DOI: 10.1186/s13000-019-0891-4

[95] Leung S, Liu X, Fang L, et al. The cytokine milieu in the interplay of pathogenic Th1/Th17 cells and regulatory T cells in autoimmune disease. Cellular & Molecular Immunology. 2010;**7**:182-189. DOI: 10.1038/cmi.2010.22

[96] Lee J, Lozano-Ruiz B, Yang FM, et al. The multifaceted role of Th1, Th9, and Th17 cells in immune checkpoint inhibition therapy. Frontiers in Immunology. 2021;**12**. DOI: 10.3389/fimmu.2021.625667

[97] Blaschitz C, Raffatellu M. Th17 cytokines and the gut mucosal barrier. Journal of Clinical Immunology. 2010; **30**:196-203. DOI: 10.1007/s10875-010-9368-7

[98] Lee Jacob S, Tato Cristina M, Joyce-Shaikh B, et al. Interleukin-23-independent IL-17 production regulates intestinal epithelial permeability. Immunity. 2015;**43**:727-738. DOI: 10.1016/j.immuni.2015.09.003

[99] Song X. Intestinal microbiota mining: A Th17/Treg cell perspective. European Journal of BioMedical Research. 2015;**1**:28. DOI: 10.18088/ejbmr.1.4.2015.pp28-35

[100] Cheng N-C, Guan CW, et al. The Th17/Treg cell balance: A gut microbiota-modulated story. Microorganisms. 2019;7:583. DOI: 10.3390/microorganisms7120583

[101] Shao L, Li M, Zhang B, et al. Bacterial dysbiosis incites Th17 cell revolt in irradiated gut. Biomedicine & Pharmacotherapy. 2020;**131**:110674. DOI: 10.1016/j.biopha.2020.110674

[102] Pandiyan P, Bhaskaran N, Zou M, et al. Microbiome dependent regulation of Tregs and Th17 cells in mucosa. Frontiers in Immunology. 2019:**10**:426. DOI: 10.3389/fimmu.2019.00426

[103] Kang L, Fang X, Song YH, et al. Neutrophil-epithelial crosstalk during intestinal inflammation. Cellular and Molecular Gastroenterology and Hepatology. 2022;**14**:1257-1267. DOI: 10.1016/j.jcmgh.2022.09.002

[104] Kimura A, Kishimoto T. IL-6: Regulator of Treg/Th17 balance. European Journal of Immunology. 2010; **40**:1830-1835. DOI: 10.1002/eji.201040391

[105] Iebba V, Guerrieri F, Di Gregorio V, et al. Combining amplicon sequencing and metabolomics in cirrhotic patients highlights distinctive microbiota features involved in bacterial translocation, systemic inflammation and hepatic encephalopathy. Scientific Reports. 2018;**8**:8210. DOI: 10.1038/s41598-018-26509-y

[106] Manzhalii E, Virchenko O, Falalyeyeva T, et al. Hepatic encephalopathy aggravated by systemic inflammation. Digestive Diseases. 2019; **37**:509-517. DOI: 10.1159/000500717

[107] Shawcross DL, Sharifi Y, Canavan JB, et al. Infection and systemic inflammation, not ammonia, are associated with grade 3/4 hepatic encephalopathy, but not mortality in cirrhosis. Journal of Hepatology. 2011;**54**: 640-649. DOI: 10.1016/j.jhep.2010.07.045

[108] Verma N, Dhiman RK, Choudhury A, et al. Dynamic assessments of hepatic encephalopathy and ammonia levels predict mortality in acute-on-chronic liver failure. Hepatology International. 2021;**15**: 970-982. DOI: 10.1007/s12072-021-10221-7

[109] Nielsen MC, Andersen MN, Rittig N, et al. The macrophage-related biomarkers sCD163 and sCD206 are released by different shedding mechanisms. Journal of Leukocyte Biology. 2019;**106**:1129-1138. DOI: 10.1002/JLB.3A1218-500R

[110] Grønbæk H, Rødgaard-Hansen S, Aagaard NK, et al. Macrophage activation markers predict mortality in patients with liver cirrhosis without or with acute-on-chronic liver failure (ACLF). Journal of Hepatology. 2016;**64**: 813-822. DOI: 10.1016/j.jhep.2015.11.021

[111] Dixon LJ, Barnes M, Tang H, et al. Kupffer cells in the liver. Comprehensive Physiology. 2013;**3**:785

[112] Ma Y-y, Yang M-q, He Z-g, et al. The Biological Function of Kupffer Cells in Liver Disease. London, UK, London, UK: IntechOpen; 2017

[113] Gomez Perdiguero E, Klapproth K, Schulz C, et al. Tissue-resident macrophages originate from yolk-sac-derived erythro-myeloid progenitors. Nature. 2015;**518**:547-551

[114] Naito M, Hasegawa G, Ebe Y, et al. Differentiation and function of Kupffer cells. Medical Electron Microscopy. 2004;**37**:16-28

[115] Scott CL, Zheng F, De Baetselier P, et al. Bone marrow-derived monocytes give rise to self-renewing and fully differentiated Kupffer cells. Nature Communications. 2016;**7**:10321. DOI: 10.1038/ncomms10321

[116] Laskin DL, Sunil VR, Gardner CR, et al. Macrophages and tissue injury: Agents of defense or destruction? Annual Review of Pharmacology and Toxicology. 2011;**51**:267-288

[117] Sica A, Mantovani A. Macrophage plasticity and polarization: *In vivo* veritas. The Journal of Clinical Investigation. 2012;**122**:787-795

[118] Sato K, Hall C, Glaser S, et al. Pathogenesis of Kupffer cells in cholestatic liver injury. The American Journal of Pathology. 2016;**186**: 2238-2247. DOI: 10.1016/j.ajpath.2016.06.003

[119] Weston CJ, Zimmermann HW, Adams DH. The role of myeloid-derived cells in the progression of liver disease. Frontiers in Immunology. 2019;**10**:893. DOI: 10.3389/fimmu.2019.00893

[120] An P, Wei LL, Zhao S, et al. Hepatocyte mitochondria-derived danger signals directly activate hepatic stellate cells and drive progression of liver fibrosis. Nature Communications. 2020;**11**:2362. DOI: 10.1038/s41467-020-16092-0

[121] Méndez-Sánchez N, Valencia-Rodríguez A, Coronel-Castillo C, et al. The cellular pathways of liver fibrosis in non-alcoholic steatohepatitis. Annals of Translational Medicine. 2020;**8**:400

[122] Yan Y, Zeng J, Xing L, et al. Extra- and intra-cellular mechanisms of hepatic stellate cell activation. Biomedicine. 2021;**9**:1014. DOI: 10.3390/biomedicines9081014

[123] Weiskirchen R, Tacke F. Cellular and molecular functions of hepatic stellate cells in inflammatory responses and liver immunology. Hepatobiliary Surgery and Nutrition. 2014;**3**:344-363

[124] Brass A, Brenndörfer ED. The role of chemokines in hepatitis C virus-mediated liver disease. International Journal of Molecular Sciences. 2014;**15**:4747-4779. DOI: 10.3390/ijms15034747

[125] Nishikawa K, Osawa Y, Kimura K. Wnt/β-catenin signaling as a potential target for the treatment of liver cirrhosis using antifibrotic drugs. International Journal of Molecular Sciences. 2018;**19**:3103

[126] Xu F, Liu C, Zhou D, et al. TGF-β/SMAD pathway and its regulation in hepatic fibrosis. Journal of Histochemistry & Cytochemistry. 2016;**64**:157-167

[127] Inzaugarat ME, Johnson CD, Holtmann TM, et al. NLR family pyrin domain-containing 3 inflammasome activation in hepatic stellate cells induces liver fibrosis in mice. Hepatology. 2019;**69**:845-859. DOI: 10.1002/hep.30252

[128] Gao B, Jeong W-I, Tian Z. Liver: An organ with predominant innate immunity. Hepatology. 2008;**47**:729-736

[129] Su GL, Klein RD, Aminlari A, et al. Kupffer cell activation by lipopolysaccharide in rats: Role for lipopolysaccharide binding protein and toll-like receptor 4. Hepatology. 2000;**31**:932-936

[130] Jia F, Deng F, Xu P, et al. NOD1 agonist protects against lipopolysaccharide and D-galactosamine-induced fatal hepatitis through the upregulation of A20 expression in hepatocytes. Frontiers in Immunology. 2021;**12**:603192. DOI: 10.3389/fimmu.2021.603192

[131] Su GL. Lipopolysaccharides in liver injury: Molecular mechanisms of Kupffer cell activation. American Journal of Physiology-Gastrointestinal and Liver Physiology. 2002;**283**:G256-G265

[132] Fisher JE, McKenzie TJ, Lillegard JB, et al. Role of Kupffer cells and toll-like receptor 4 in acetaminophen-induced acute liver failure. The Journal of Surgical Research. 2013;**180**:147-155. DOI: 10.1016/j.jss.2012.11.051

[133] Seki E, Tsutsui H, Nakano H, et al. Lipopolysaccharide-induced IL-18 secretion from murine Kupffer cells independently of myeloid differentiation factor 88 that is critically involved in induction of production of IL-12 and IL-1β. The Journal of Immunology. 2001;**166**:2651-2657

[134] Werner M, Schefczyk S, Trippler M, et al. Antiviral toll-like receptor signaling in non-parenchymal liver cells is restricted to TLR3. Viruses. 2022;**14**:218

[135] van der Heide D, Weiskirchen R, Bansal R. Therapeutic targeting of hepatic macrophages for the treatment of liver diseases. Frontiers in Immunology. 2019;**10**:2852. DOI: 10.3389/fimmu.2019.02852

[136] Faruqui A. Alcohol induced gut microbiota modulation: The role of probiotics, pufas, and vitamin E in management of alcoholic liver disease, Japanese. Journal of Gastroenterology and Hepatology. 2021;**5**:1-9. DOI: 10.47829/JJGH.2021.51304

[137] Dong X, Liu J, Xu Y, et al. Role of macrophages in experimental liver injury and repair in mice (review). Experimental and Therapeutic Medicine. 2019;**17**:3835-3847. DOI: 10.3892/etm.2019.7450

[138] Heath WR, Carbone FR. Dendritic cell subsets in primary and secondary T cell responses at body surfaces. Nature Immunology. 2009;**10**:1237-1244

[139] Henri S, Guilliams M, Poulin LF, et al. Disentangling the complexity of the skin dendritic cell network. Immunology & Cell Biology. 2010;**88**:366-375. DOI: 10.1038/icb.2010.34

[140] Guilliams M, Henri S, Tamoutounour S, et al. From skin dendritic cells to a simplified classification of human and mouse dendritic cell subsets. European Journal of Immunology. 2010;**40**:2089-2094. DOI: 10.1002/eji.201040498

[141] Manh TP, Alexandre Y, Baranek T, et al. Plasmacytoid, conventional, and monocyte-derived dendritic cells undergo a profound and convergent genetic reprogramming during their maturation. European Journal of Immunology. 2013;**43**:1706-1715. DOI: 10.1002/eji.201243106

[142] Zhang Z, Zou Z-S, Fu J-L, et al. Severe dendritic cell perturbation is actively involved in the pathogenesis of acute-on-chronic hepatitis B liver failure. Journal of Hepatology. 2008;**49**: 396-406. DOI: 10.1016/j.jhep.2008.05.017

[143] Khanam A, Trehanpati N, Garg V, et al. Altered frequencies of dendritic cells and IFN-γ-secreting T cells with granulocyte colony-stimulating factor (G-CSF) therapy in acute-on-chronic liver failure. Liver International. 2014;**34**: 505-513

[144] Edwards AD, Diebold SS, Slack EM, et al. Toll-like receptor expression in murine DC subsets: Lack of TLR7 expression by CD8 alpha+ DC correlates with unresponsiveness to imidazoquinolines. European Journal of Immunology. 2003;**33**:827-833. DOI: 10.1002/eji.200323797

[145] Cervantes JL, Weinerman B, Basole C, et al. TLR8: The forgotten relative revindicated. Cellular & Molecular Immunology. 2012;**9**:434-438. DOI: 10.1038/cmi.2012.38

[146] Sundar R, Cho B-C, Brahmer J, et al. Nivolumab in NSCLC: Latest evidence and clinical potential. Therapeutic Advances in Medical Oncology. 2015;**7**:85-96. DOI: 10.1177/1758834014567470

[147] Helft J, Ginhoux F, Bogunovic M, et al. Origin and functional heterogeneity of non-lymphoid tissue dendritic cells in mice. Immunological Reviews. 2010;**234**:55-75

[148] Kumar J, Habib N, Huang K-W, et al. Recent advances: The imbalance of immune cells and cytokines in the pathogenesis of hepatocellular carcinoma. Diagnostics (Basel). 2020;**10**: 338. DOI: 10.3390/diagnostics10050338

[149] Sutti S, Bruzzì S, Heymann F, et al. CX3CR1 mediates the development of monocyte-derived dendritic cells during hepatic inflammation. Cell. 2019;**8**:1099. DOI: 10.3390/cells8091099

[150] Chang Q, Wang Y-K, Zhao Q, et al. Th17 cells are increased with severity of liver inflammation in patients with chronic hepatitis C. Journal of Gastroenterology and Hepatology. 2012; **27**:273-278. DOI: 10.1111/j.1440-1746.2011.06782.x

[151] Sun HQ, Zhang JY, Zhang H, et al. Increased Th17 cells contribute to disease progression in patients with HBV-associated liver cirrhosis. Journal of Viral Hepatitis. 2012;**19**:396-403. DOI: 10.1111/j.1365-2893.2011.01561.x

[152] Mou H, Wu S, Zhao G, et al. Changes of Th17/Treg ratio in the transition of chronic hepatitis B to liver cirrhosis and correlations with liver function and inflammation. Experimental and Therapeutic Medicine. 2019;**17**:2963-2968. DOI: 10.3892/etm.2019.7299

[153] Zepeda-Morales AS, Del Toro-Arreola S, García-Benavides L, et al. Liver fibrosis in bile duct-ligated rats correlates with increased hepatic IL-17 and TGF-β2 expression. Annals of Hepatology. 2016;**15**:418-426. DOI: 10.5604/16652681.1198820

[154] Luckey SW, Petersen DR. Activation of Kupffer cells during the course of carbon tetrachloride-induced liver injury and fibrosis in rats. Experimental and Molecular Pathology. 2001;**71**:226-240. DOI: 10.1006/exmp.2001.2399

[155] Aoyama T, Inokuchi S, Brenner DA, et al. CX3CL1-CX3CR1 interaction prevents carbon tetrachloride-induced liver inflammation and fibrosis in mice. Hepatology. 2010;**52**:1390-1400. DOI: 10.1002/hep.23795

[156] Dhanda S, Gupta S, Halder A, et al. Systemic inflammation without gliosis mediates cognitive deficits through impaired BDNF expression in bile duct ligation model of hepatic encephalopathy. Brain, Behavior, and Immunity. 2018;**70**:214-232. DOI: 10.1016/j.bbi.2018.03.002

[157] Tung HC, Lee FY, Wang SS, et al. The beneficial effects of P2X7 antagonism in rats with bile duct ligation-induced cirrhosis. PLoS One. 2015;**10**:e0124654. DOI: 10.1371/journal.pone.0124654

[158] Kang H, Koppula S. Hepatoprotective effect of houttuynia cordata thunb extract against carbon tetrachloride-induced hepatic damage in mice. Indian Journal of Pharmaceutical Sciences. 2014;**76**:267-273

[159] Moles A, Murphy L, Wilson CL, et al. A TLR2/S100A9/CXCL-2 signaling network is necessary for neutrophil recruitment in acute and chronic liver injury in the mouse. Journal of Hepatology. 2014;**60**: 782-791. DOI: 10.1016/j.jhep.2013.12.005

[160] Altaş S, Kızıl G, Kızıl M, et al. Protective effect of Diyarbakır watermelon juice on carbon tetrachloride-induced toxicity in rats. Food and Chemical Toxicology. 2011;**49**: 2433-2438. DOI: 10.1016/j.fct.2011.06.064

[161] Tag CG, Sauer-Lehnen S, Weiskirchen S, et al. Bile duct ligation in mice: Induction of inflammatory liver injury and fibrosis by obstructive cholestasis. Journal of Visualized Experiments. 2015;**96**:52438. DOI: 10.3791/52438

[162] Canbay A, Feldstein A, Baskin-Bey E, et al. The caspase inhibitor IDN-6556 attenuates hepatic injury and fibrosis in the bile duct ligated mouse. Journal of Pharmacology and Experimental Therapeutics. 2004;**308**:1191-1196. DOI: 10.1124/jpet.103.060129

[163] Trebicka J, Hennenberg M, Odenthal M, et al. Atorvastatin attenuates hepatic fibrosis in rats after bile duct ligation via decreased turnover of hepatic stellate cells. Journal of Hepatology. 2010;**53**:702-712. DOI: 10.1016/j.jhep.2010.04.025

[164] Gobejishvili L, Barve S, Breitkopf-Heinlein K, et al. Rolipram attenuates bile duct ligation–induced liver injury in rats: A potential pathogenic role of PDE4. Journal of Pharmacology and Experimental Therapeutics. 2013;**347**: 80-90. DOI: 10.1124/jpet.113.204933

[165] Weng Z, Chi Y, Xie J, et al. Anti-inflammatory activity of dehydroandrographolide by TLR4/NF-κB signaling pathway inhibition in bile duct-ligated mice. Cellular Physiology and Biochemistry. 2018;**49**:1124-1137. DOI: 10.1159/000493292

[166] Gehring S, Dickson EM, San Martin ME, et al. Kupffer cells abrogate cholestatic liver injury in mice. Gastroenterology. 2006;**130**:810-822. DOI: 10.1053/j.gastro.2005.11.015

[167] Alric L, Orfila C, Carrere N, et al. Reactive oxygen intermediates and eicosanoid production by Kupffer cells and infiltrated macrophages in acute and chronic liver injury induced in rats by CCl4. Inflammation Research. 2000;**49**: 700-707. DOI: 10.1007/s000110050649

[168] Nagano T, Yamamoto K, Matsumoto S, et al. Cytokine profile in the liver of primary biliary cirrhosis. Journal of Clinical Immunology. 1999; **19**:422-427. DOI: 10.1023/A:1020511 002025

[169] Holland-Fischer P, Grønbæk H, Sandahl TD, et al. Kupffer cells are activated in cirrhotic portal hypertension and not normalised by TIPS. Gut. 2011; **60**:1389-1393. DOI: 10.1136/ gut.2010.234542

[170] de Lalla C, Galli G, Aldrighetti L, et al. Production of profibrotic cytokines by invariant NKT cells characterizes cirrhosis progression in chronic viral Hepatitis1. The Journal of Immunology. 2004;**173**:1417-1425. DOI: 10.4049/ jimmunol.173.2.1417

[171] Napoli J, Bishop GA, McGuinness PH, et al. Progressive liver injury in chronic hepatitis C infection correlates with increased intrahepatic expression of Th1-associated cytokines. Hepatology. 1996;**24**:759-765. DOI: 10.1002/hep.510240402

[172] Farinati F, Cardin R, Bortolami M, et al. Oxidative damage, pro-inflammatory cytokines, TGF-alpha and c-myc in chronic HCV-related hepatitis and cirrhosis. World Journal of Gastroenterology. 2006;**12**:2065-2069. DOI: 10.3748/wjg.v12.i13.2065

[173] Li H, Xia Q, Zeng B, et al. Submassive hepatic necrosis distinguishes HBV-associated acute on chronic liver failure from cirrhotic patients with acute decompensation. Journal of Hepatology. 2015;**63**:50-59. DOI: 10.1016/j.jhep.2015.01.029

[174] Chuang Y-H, Lian Z-X, Tsuneyama K, et al. Increased killing activity and decreased cytokine production in NK cells in patients with primary biliary cirrhosis. Journal of Autoimmunity. 2006;**26**:232-240. DOI: 10.1016/j.jaut.2006.04.001

[175] Schafer DP, Stevens B. Microglia function in central nervous system development and plasticity. Cold Spring Harbor Perspectives in Biology. 2015;7: a020545. DOI: 10.1101/cshperspect. a020545

[176] Fujita Y, Yamashita T. Neuroprotective function of microglia in the developing brain. Neuronal Signaling. 2021;**5**:Ns20200024. DOI: 10.1042/ns20200024

[177] Wolf SA, Boddeke HW, Kettenmann H. Microglia in physiology and disease. Annual Review of Physiology. 2017;**79**:619-643. DOI: 10.1146/annurev-physiol-022516-034406

[178] Wlodarczyk A, Løbner M, Cédile O, et al. Comparison of microglia and infiltrating CD11c+ cells as antigen presenting cells for T cell proliferation and cytokine response. Journal of Neuroinflammation. 2014;**11**:1-9

[179] Borst K, Dumas AA, Prinz M. Microglia: Immune and non-immune functions. Immunity. 2021;**54**:2194-2208

[180] Hsieh CL, Koike M, Spusta SC, et al. A role for TREM2 ligands in the phagocytosis of apoptotic neuronal cells by microglia. Journal of Neurochemistry. 2009;**109**:1144-1156

[181] Takahashi K, Rochford CD, Neumann H. Clearance of apoptotic neurons without inflammation by microglial triggering receptor expressed on myeloid cells-2. The Journal of Experimental Medicine. 2005;**201**: 647-657

[182] Wu D, Chen Q, Chen X, et al. The blood–brain barrier: Structure, regulation, and drug delivery. Signal Transduction and Targeted Therapy. 2023;**8**:217. DOI: 10.1038/s41392-023-01481-w

[183] Lochhead JJ, Yang J, Ronaldson PT, et al. Structure, function, and regulation of the blood-brain barrier tight junction in central nervous system disorders. Frontiers in Physiology. 2020;**11**:914. DOI: 10.3389/fphys.2020.00914

[184] Farooq RK, Alamoudi W, Alhibshi A, et al. Varied composition and underlying mechanisms of gut microbiome in neuroinflammation. Microorganisms. 2022;**10**:705

[185] Buttgereit A, Lelios I, Yu X, et al. Sall1 is a transcriptional regulator defining microglia identity and function. Nature Immunology. 2016;**17**:1397-1406

[186] Li K, Tan Y-H, Light AR, et al. Different peripheral tissue injury induces differential phenotypic changes of spinal activated microglia. Clinical and Developmental Immunology. 2013; **2013**:901420

[187] Brockie S, Hong J, Fehlings MG. The role of microglia in modulating neuroinflammation after spinal cord injury. International Journal of Molecular Sciences. 2021;**22**:9706

[188] Ohsawa K, Imai Y, Sasaki Y, et al. Microglia/macrophage-specific protein Iba1 binds to fimbrin and enhances its actin-bundling activity. Journal of Neurochemistry. 2004;**88**:844-856. DOI: 10.1046/j.1471-4159.2003.02213.x

[189] Fadini GP, Cappellari R, Mazzucato M, et al. Monocyte–

macrophage polarization balance in prediabetic individuals. Acta Diabetologica. 2013;**50**:977-982

[190] Jones BA, Beamer M, Ahmed S. Fractalkine/CX3CL1: A potential new target for inflammatory diseases. Molecular Interventions. 2010;**10**:263

[191] Jiang SX, Slinn J, Aylsworth A, et al. Vimentin participates in microglia activation and neurotoxicity in cerebral ischemia. Journal of Neurochemistry. 2012;**122**:764-774. DOI: 10.1111/j.1471-4159.2012.07823.x

[192] Masuda T, Amann L, Sankowski R, et al. Novel Hexb-based tools for studying microglia in the CNS. Nature Immunology. 2020;**21**:802-815. DOI: 10.1038/s41590-020-0707-4

[193] Leyh J, Paeschke S, Mages B, et al. Classification of microglial morphological phenotypes using machine learning. Frontiers in Cellular Neuroscience. 2021;**15**:701673. DOI: 10.3389/fncel.2021.701673

[194] Vidal-Itriago A, Radford RAW, Aramideh JA, et al. Microglia morphophysiological diversity and its implications for the CNS. Frontiers in Immunology. 2022;**13**:997786. DOI: 10.3389/fimmu.2022.997786

[195] Davalos D, Grutzendler J, Yang G, et al. ATP mediates rapid microglial response to local brain injury *in vivo*. Nature Neuroscience. 2005;**8**:752-758. DOI: 10.1038/nn1472

[196] Das Sarma S, Chatterjee K, Dinda H, et al. Cytomorphological and cytochemical identification of microglia. International Scholarly Research Notices. 2013;**2013**:205431

[197] Borch J, Haslund-Vinding J, Vilhardt F, et al. Meningioma–brain crosstalk: A scoping review. Cancers. 2021;**13**:4267. DOI: 10.3390/cancers13174267

[198] Jurga AM, Paleczna M, Kuter KZ. Overview of general and discriminating markers of differential microglia phenotypes. Frontiers in Cellular Neuroscience. 2020;**14**:198. DOI: 10.3389/fncel.2020.00198

[199] Rodrigo R, Cauli O, Gomez–Pinedo U et al. Hyperammonemia induces neuroinflammation that contributes to cognitive impairment in rats with hepatic encephalopathy, Gastroenterology 2010;139:675-684. doi: 10.1053/j.gastro.2010.03.040.

[200] Tamnanloo F, Ochoa-Sanchez R, Oliveira MM, et al. Multiple ammonia-induced episodes of hepatic encephalopathy provoke neuronal cell loss in bile-duct ligated rats. JHEP Reports. 2023;**5**:100904. DOI: 10.1016/j.jhepr.2023.100904

[201] Bosoi CR, Yang X, Huynh J, et al. Systemic oxidative stress is implicated in the pathogenesis of brain edema in rats with chronic liver failure. Free Radical Biology and Medicine. 2012;**52**:1228-1235. DOI: 10.1016/j.freeradbiomed.2012.01.006

[202] Magen I, Avraham Y, Ackerman Z, et al. Cannabidiol ameliorates cognitive and motor impairments in mice with bile duct ligation. Journal of Hepatology. 2009;**51**:528-534. DOI: 10.1016/j.jhep.2009.04.021

[203] Clément M-A, Bosoi CR, Oliveira MM, et al. Bile-duct ligation renders the brain susceptible to hypotension-induced neuronal degeneration: Implications of ammonia. Journal of Neurochemistry. 2021;**157**:561-573. DOI: 10.1111/jnc.15290

[204] Stojanović NM, Maslovarić A, Mihajlović I, et al. Melatonin treatment prevents carbon-tetrachloride induced rat brain injury. Toxicology Research. 2023;**12**(5):895-901. DOI: 10.1093/toxres/tfad083

[205] Dhanda S, Sandhir R. Blood-brain barrier permeability is exacerbated in experimental model of hepatic encephalopathy via MMP-9 activation and downregulation of tight junction proteins. Molecular Neurobiology. 2018; **55**:3642-3659. DOI: 10.1007/s12035-017-0521-7

[206] Yang N, Liu H, Jiang Y, et al. Lactulose enhances neuroplasticity to improve cognitive function in early hepatic encephalopathy. Neural Regeneration Research. 2015;**10**: 1457-1462. DOI: 10.4103/1673-5374.165516

[207] Golshani M, Basiri M, Shabani M, et al. Effects of erythropoietin on bile duct ligation-induced neuro-inflammation in male rats. AIMS Neuroscience. 2019;**6**:43-53. DOI: 10.3934/Neuroscience.2019.2.43

[208] Hsu S-J, Zhang C, Jeong J, et al. Enhanced meningeal lymphatic drainage ameliorates neuroinflammation and hepatic encephalopathy in cirrhotic rats. Gastroenterology. 2021;**160**:1315-1329. e1313. DOI: 10.1053/j.gastro.2020.11.036

[209] Chen J-R, Wang B-N, Tseng G-F, et al. Morphological changes of cortical pyramidal neurons in hepatic encephalopathy. BMC Neuroscience. 2014;**15**:15. DOI: 10.1186/1471-2202-15-15

[210] Chen Y-C, Sheen J-M, Tain Y-L, et al. Alterations in NADPH oxidase expression and blood–brain barrier in bile duct ligation-treated young rats: Effects of melatonin. Neurochemistry International. 2012;**60**:751-758. DOI: 10.1016/j.neuint.2012.03.021

[211] Pierzchala K, Simicic D, Sienkiewicz A, et al. Central nervous system and systemic oxidative stress interplay with inflammation in a bile duct ligation rat model of type C hepatic encephalopathy. Free Radical Biology and Medicine. 2022;**178**:295-307. DOI: 10.1016/j.freeradbiomed.2021.12.011

[212] Ahmadi S, Khaledi S. Anxiety in rats with bile duct ligation is associated with activation of JNK3 mitogen-activated protein kinase in the hippocampus. Metabolic Brain Disease. 2020;**35**: 579-588. DOI: 10.1007/s11011-020-00542-1

[213] Magen I, Avraham Y, Ackerman Z, et al. Cannabidiol ameliorates cognitive and motor impairments in bile-duct ligated mice via 5-HT1A receptor activation. British Journal of Pharmacology. 2010;**159**:950-957. DOI: 10.1111/j.1476-5381.2009.00589.x

[214] Gee LMV, Barron-Millar B, Leslie J, et al. Anti–cholestatic therapy with obeticholic acid improves short-term memory in bile duct–ligated mice. The American Journal of Pathology. 2023; **193**:11-26. DOI: 10.1016/j.ajpath.2022.09.005

[215] Shabani M, Ebrahimpoor F, Firouzjaei MA, et al. Modulation of sphingosine-1-phosphate receptor by FTY720 contributes in improvement of hepatic encephalopathy induced by bile duct ligation. Brain Research Bulletin. 2019;**146**:253-269. DOI: 10.1016/j.brainresbull.2019.01.012

[216] Balasubramaniyan V, Wright G, Sharma V, et al. Ammonia reduction with ornithine phenylacetate restores brain eNOS activity via the DDAH-

ADMA pathway in bile duct-ligated cirrhotic rats. American Journal of Physiology-Gastrointestinal and Liver Physiology. 2012;**302**:G145-G152. DOI: 10.1152/ajpgi.00097.2011

[217] Wright G, Wright G, Newman T, et al. OP08 evidence for early astrocyte activation, cellular stress and compensatory microglial related transforming growth factor-α responses in bile-duct ligated rats. Gut. 2010;**59**: A3-A4. DOI: 10.1136/gut.2010.223362.8

[218] Faropoulos K, Chroni E, Assimakopoulos SF, et al. Altered occludin expression in brain capillaries induced by obstructive jaundice in rats. Brain Research. 2010;**1325**:121-127. DOI: 10.1016/j.brainres.2010.02.020

[219] Boer LA, Panatto JP, Fagundes DA, et al. Inhibition of mitochondrial respiratory chain in the brain of rats after hepatic failure induced by carbon tetrachloride is reversed by antioxidants. Brain Research Bulletin. 2009;**80**:75-78. DOI: 10.1016/j.brainresbull.2009.04.009

[220] Khan A, Shal B, Naveed M, et al. Matrine ameliorates anxiety and depression-like behaviour by targeting hyperammonemia-induced neuroinflammation and oxidative stress in CCl4 model of liver injury. Neurotoxicology. 2019;**72**:38-50. DOI: 10.1016/j.neuro.2019.02.002

[221] de Souza MF, Marinho JP, Abujamra AL, et al. Carbon tetrachloride increases the pro-inflammatory cytokines levels in different brain areas of Wistar rats: The protective effect of acai frozen pulp. Neurochemical Research. 2015;**40**:1976-1983. DOI: 10.1007/s11064-015-1693-z

[222] Hadjihambi A, Harrison IF, Costas-Rodríguez M, et al. Impaired brain glymphatic flow in experimental hepatic encephalopathy. Journal of Hepatology. 2019;**70**:40-49. DOI: 10.1016/j.jhep.2018.08.021

[223] Zemtsova I, Görg B, Keitel V, et al. Microglia activation in hepatic encephalopathy in rats and humans. Hepatology. 2011;**54**:204-215. DOI: 10.1002/hep.24326

[224] Görg B, Bidmon H-J, Häussinger D. Gene expression profiling in the cerebral cortex of patients with cirrhosis with and without hepatic encephalopathy. Hepatology. 2013;**57**:2436-2447

[225] Grover VPB, Pavese N, Koh S-B, et al. Cerebral microglial activation in patients with hepatitis C: *In vivo* evidence of neuroinflammation. Journal of Viral Hepatitis. 2012;**19**:e89-e96. DOI: 10.1111/j.1365-2893.2011.01510.x

[226] Balzano T, Forteza J, Molina P, et al. The cerebellum of patients with steatohepatitis shows lymphocyte infiltration, microglial activation and loss of Purkinje and granular neurons. Scientific Reports. 2018;**8**:3004. DOI: 10.1038/s41598-018-21399-6

[227] Cagnin A, Taylor-Robinson SD, Forton DM, et al. In vivo imaging of cerebral "peripheral benzodiazepine binding sites" in patients with hepatic encephalopathy. Gut. 2006;**55**:547. DOI: 10.1136/gut.2005.075051

[228] Butterworth RF, Lavoie J, Giguère J-F, et al. Affinities and densities of high-affinity [3H]muscimol (GABA-A) binding sites and of central benzodiazepine receptors are unchanged in autopsied brain tissue from cirrhotic patients with hepatic encephalopathy. Hepatology. 1988;**8**:1084-1088. DOI: 10.1002/hep.1840080517

[229] Milewski K, Orzeł-Gajowik K, Zielińska M. Mitochondrial changes in

rat brain endothelial cells associated with hepatic encephalopathy: Relation to the blood–brain barrier dysfunction. Neurochemical Research. 2022. pp.1-16. DOI: 10.1007/s11064-022-03698-7

[230] Claeys W, Van Hoecke L, Lefere S, et al. The neurogliovascular unit in hepatic encephalopathy. JHEP Reports. 2021;**3**:100352. DOI: 10.1016/j.jhepr.2021.100352

[231] Linnerbauer M, Wheeler MA, Quintana FJ. Astrocyte crosstalk in CNS inflammation. Neuron. 2020;**108**: 608-622

[232] Ede RJ, Zaki AEO, Silk DBA, et al. Experimental studies of blood-brain barrier permeability in chronic hepatic encephalopathy. In: Advances in Hepatic Encephalopathy and Urea Cycle Diseases: 5th International Symposium on Ammonia, Semmering, Austria, Basel, Switzerland. May 1984: Proceedings. S. Karger AG; 1985

[233] Vairappan B, Sundhar M, Srinivas BH. Resveratrol restores neuronal tight junction proteins through correction of ammonia and inflammation in CCl(4)-induced cirrhotic mice. Molecular Neurobiology. 2019;**56**:4718-4729. DOI: 10.1007/s12035-018-1389-x

[234] Baek SY, Lee EH, Oh TW, et al. Network pharmacology-based approaches of rheum undulatum linne and glycyrriza uralensis fischer imply their regulation of liver failure with hepatic encephalopathy in mice. Biomolecules. 2020;**10**:437

[235] Quinn M, McMillin M, Galindo C, et al. Bile acids permeabilize the blood brain barrier after bile duct ligation in rats via Rac1-dependent mechanisms. Digestive and Liver Disease. 2014;**46**: 527-534. DOI: 10.1016/j.dld.2014.01.159

[236] Ott P, Larsen FS. Blood–brain barrier permeability to ammonia in liver failure: A critical reappraisal. Neurochemistry International. 2004;**44**: 185-198. DOI: 10.1016/S0197-0186(03)00153-0

[237] Chesler M. Regulation and modulation of pH in the brain. Physiological Reviews. 2003;**83**: 1183-1221

[238] Hertz L, Peng L, Song D. Ammonia, like K+, stimulates the Na+, K+, 2 Cl– cotransporter NKCC1 and the Na+, K+-ATPase and interacts with endogenous ouabain in astrocytes. Neurochemical Research. 2015;**40**:241-257

[239] Larsen EH, Deaton LE, Onken H, et al. Osmoregulation and excretion. Comprehensive Physiology. 2011;**4**: 405-573

[240] Adlimoghaddam A, Ml B, Marini A-M, et al. Ammonia excretion in *Caenorhabditis elegans*: Mechanism and evidence of ammonia transport of the rhesus protein CeRhr-1. The Journal of Experimental Biology. 2015;**218**: 675-683

[241] Watkins LR, Maier SF, Goehler LE. Cytokine-to-brain communication: A review & analysis of alternative mechanisms. Life Sciences. 1995;**57**: 1011-1026. DOI: 10.1016/0024-3205(95)02047-m

[242] D'Mello C, Swain MG. Immune-to-brain communication pathways in inflammation-associated sickness and depression. Current Topics in Behavioral Neurosciences. 2017;**31**:73-94. DOI: 10.1007/7854_2016_37

[243] Dantzer R, O'connor JC, Freund GG, et al. From inflammation to sickness and depression: When the

immune system subjugates the brain. Nature Reviews Neuroscience. 2008;**9**: 46-56

[244] Ganong WF. Circumventricular organs: Definition and role in the regulation of endocrine and autonomic function. Clinical and Experimental Pharmacology & Physiology. 2000;**27**: 422-427. DOI: 10.1046/j.1440-1681.2000.03259.x

[245] Jaeger V, DeMorrow S, McMillin M. The direct contribution of astrocytes and microglia to the pathogenesis of hepatic encephalopathy. Journal of Clinical and Translational Hepatology. 2019;**7**:352-361. DOI: 10.14218/jcth.2019.00025

[246] Garden GA, Möller T. Microglia biology in health and disease. Journal of Neuroimmune Pharmacology. 2006;**1**: 127-137

[247] Butterworth RF. Hepatic encephalopathy: A central neuroinflammatory disorder? Hepatology. 2011;**53**:1372-1376

[248] Wright GA, Sharifi Y, Newman TA, et al. Characterisation of temporal microglia and astrocyte immune responses in bile duct-ligated rat models of cirrhosis. Liver International. 2014;**34**: 1184-1191

[249] Rao KVR, Brahmbhatt M, Norenberg MD. Microglia contribute to ammonia-induced astrocyte swelling in culture. Metabolic Brain Disease. 2013; **28**:139-143

[250] Karababa A, Groos-Sahr K, Albrecht U, et al. Ammonia attenuates LPS-induced upregulation of pro-inflammatory cytokine mRNA in co-cultured astrocytes and microglia. Neurochemical Research. 2017;**42**: 737-749

[251] Fukushima S, Furube E, Itoh M, et al. Robust increase of microglia proliferation in the fornix of hippocampal axonal pathway after a single LPS stimulation. Journal of Neuroimmunology. 2015;**285**:31-40. DOI: 10.1016/j.jneuroim.2015.05.014

[252] Li Y, Yin L, Fan Z, et al. Microglia: A potential therapeutic target for sepsis-associated encephalopathy and sepsis-associated chronic pain. Frontiers in Pharmacology. 2020;**11**:600421. DOI: 10.3389/fphar.2020.600421

[253] Zargar S, Wani TA. Protective role of quercetin in carbon tetrachloride induced toxicity in rat brain: Biochemical, spectrophotometric assays and computational approach. Molecules. 2021;**26**:7526. DOI: 10.3390/molecules26247526

[254] Kim E, Cho S. Microglia and monocyte-derived macrophages in stroke. Neurotherapeutics. 2016;**13**: 702-718. DOI: 10.1007/s13311-016-0463-1

[255] Somebang K, Rudolph J, Imhof I, et al. CCR2 deficiency alters activation of microglia subsets in traumatic brain injury. Cell Reports. 2021;**36**:109727. DOI: 10.1016/j.celrep.2021.109727

[256] D'Mello C, Le T, Swain MG. Cerebral microglia recruit monocytes into the brain in response to tumor necrosis factorα signaling during peripheral organ inflammation. The Journal of Neuroscience. 2009;**29**: 2089-2102. DOI: 10.1523/jneurosci.3567-08.2009

[257] Carlos P-M, Aldo T-D. Astrocyte pathophysiology in liver disease. In: Maria Teresa G, Luca Colucci DA, editors. Astrocyte. Rijeka: IntechOpen; 2017, Ch. 10

[258] Han W, Zhang H, Han Y, et al. Cognition-tracking-based strategies for diagnosis and treatment of minimal hepatic encephalopathy. Metabolic Brain Disease. 2020;**35**:869-881. DOI: 10.1007/s11011-020-00539-w

[259] Chen Z, Ruan J, Li D, et al. The role of intestinal bacteria and gut–brain axis in hepatic encephalopathy. Frontiers in Cellular and Infection Microbiology. 2021;**10**:595759. DOI: 10.3389/fcimb.2020.595759

[260] Sorge RE, Mapplebeck JC, Rosen S, et al. Different immune cells mediate mechanical pain hypersensitivity in male and female mice. Nature Neuroscience. 2015;**18**:1081-1083

[261] Elsherbini DMA, Ghoneim FM, El-Mancy EM, et al. Astrocytes profiling in acute hepatic encephalopathy: Possible enrolling of glial fibrillary acidic protein, tumor necrosis factor-alpha, inwardly rectifying potassium channel (Kir 4.1) and aquaporin-4 in rat cerebral cortex. Frontiers in Cellular Neuroscience. 2022;**16**:896172. DOI: 10.3389/fncel.2022.896172

[262] Córdoba J, Alonso J, Rovira A, et al. The development of low-grade cerebral edema in cirrhosis is supported by the evolution of (1)H-magnetic resonance abnormalities after liver transplantation. Journal of Hepatology. 2001;**35**:598-604. DOI: 10.1016/s0168-8278(01)00181-7

[263] Jover R, Rodrigo R, Felipo V, et al. Brain edema and inflammatory activation in bile duct ligated rats with diet-induced hyperammonemia: A model of hepatic encephalopathy in cirrhosis. Hepatology. 2006;**43**:1257-1266. DOI: 10.1002/hep.21180

[264] Sepehrinezhad A, Stolze Larsen F, Ashayeri Ahmadabad R, et al. The glymphatic system may play a vital role in the pathogenesis of hepatic encephalopathy: A narrative review. Cells. 2023;**12**:979. DOI: 10.3390/cells12070979

Chapter 6

Management of Liver Cirrhosis and Its Complications

Zhenyu Wu, Lei Chen, Jing Chen and Chuanfang Chen

Abstract

Liver cirrhosis is a widespread global health concern with various potential causes, such as chronic viral hepatitis, nonalcoholic fatty liver disease, alcohol consumption, and autoimmune diseases. The development of cirrhosis occurs over an extended period of chronic inflammation, leading to the substitution of healthy liver tissue with fibrotic tissue and regenerative nodules, ultimately leading to the onset of portal hypertension. Decompensated cirrhosis, which arises from a compensated stage, is characterized by the emergence of complications such as ascites, esophageal variceal bleeding, hepatorenal syndrome, hepatic encephalopathy, portal vein thrombosis, and hepatocellular carcinoma, which will result in prolonged hospitalization, impaired quality of life, and poor survival. In recent years, a concept known as "cirrhosis recompensation" has gained prominence in the field of liver cirrhosis. Cirrhosis recompensation, as defined by the Baveno VII consensus criteria, involves three core elements: addressing the underlying etiological factors, achieving remission from complications that are characteristic of the decompensated stage of cirrhosis, and achieving improvements in liver function. Consequently, the management of cirrhosis focuses on the elimination of underlying etiologies, surveillance for hepatocellular carcinoma and esophageal varices, assessment of suitability for liver transplantation, and treatment of complications.

Keywords: variceal bleeding, ascites, spontaneous bacterial peritonitis, encephalopathy, hepatorenal syndrome

1. Introduction

Liver cirrhosis progresses through two main stages: compensated and decompensated. As cirrhotic patients progress to the decompensated stage, they may suffer from a spectrum of complications including ascites, variceal bleeding, hepatorenal syndrome, hepatic encephalopathy, portal vein thrombosis, and hepatocellular carcinoma. Recently, experts have introduced the concept of recompensation [1, 2], where decompensated cirrhotic patients exhibit the recompensation of ascites (without the use of diuretics), absence of hepatic encephalopathy (without the use of lactulose or rifaximin), no recurrence of esophagogastric variceal bleeding (EGVB) for at least 12 months, and sustained stability of liver function parameters upon the suppression and elimination of underlying etiologies. Therefore, treatment of the underlying etiologies and complications is of paramount importance to improve patients' prognoses.

IntechOpen

The etiologies of cirrhosis encompass viral hepatitis, alcoholic liver disease (ALD), nonalcoholic fatty liver disease (NAFLD), autoimmune liver diseases, drug-induced liver injury, genetic and metabolic disorders, and hepatic vascular diseases [3, 4]. Elimination of the underlying causes is the most crucial therapeutic intervention in the management of cirrhosis. Antiviral therapy can effectively eliminate viral replication, which will delay the progression of cirrhosis and result in recompensation in some cases. Alcohol abstinence is the primary treatment strategy for alcohol-related liver cirrhosis and may lead to a shift from decompensated to compensated stage. Cirrhotic patients are advised to abstain from alcohol and smoking, irrespective of etiologies [5, 6]. With the improvement of lifestyle, nonalcoholic fatty liver disease (NAFLD), also named metabolic dysfunction-associated fatty liver disease (MAFLD), affects approximately 30% of the global population and has become the predominant cause of liver diseases worldwide. Weight loss and lifestyle improvements will decrease the incidence of NAFLD and slow down disease progression. Corticosteroids (prednisone) and immunosuppressants (azathioprine) are used as first-line treatment of autoimmune liver disease. However, incomplete elimination of the etiologies [7, 8], advanced age (> 65 years), persistent inflammatory necrotic activity in the liver pathology, and advanced cirrhosis (Child-Pugh class C, MELD score > 20, serum albumin level < 35 g/L, HVPG >16 mmHg) will contribute to non-reversal of liver fibrosis and cirrhosis even when patients receive etiological treatment.

Liver function preservation and nutritional improvement are pivotal strategies in the management of cirrhosis. Pharmacological agents for liver function preservation include glycyrrhizin preparations, silymarin, and polyenylphosphatidylcholine. Ursodeoxycholic acid and tauroursodeoxycholic acid are effective in improving intrahepatic cholestasis [9–11]. Research indicates that statin usage can slow disease progression and decrease mortality. Statins are recommended for patients classified as Child-Pugh A and B [12]. However, they are not recommended for patients with Child-Pugh C due to unclear adverse effects including hepatotoxicity and rhabdomyolysis in these cases [13]. Malnutrition is an independent risk factor for mortality in patients with decompensated cirrhosis, significantly attributed to inadequate protein intake [14]. It is currently known that plant-based proteins are superior to animal-based proteins in reducing the incidence of hepatic encephalopathy. Given the inadequate hepatic glycogen reserves, prolonged fasting can stimulate muscle glycogen mobilization and fatty acid oxidation, thereby increasing the risk of sarcopenia. Consequently, patients with cirrhosis are recommended to adopt a strategy of frequent, smaller meals, complemented by vitamins, trace elements (such as zinc), and dietary fiber supplementation. Additionally, aerobic and resistance training are highly recommended.

2. Management of esophagogastric varices

2.1 Surveillance

As liver cirrhosis progresses, influenced by angiogenic factors, numerous neovessels emerge, leading to increased hepatic blood flow. This process also stimulates the proliferation of hepatic venous tributaries [15]. Subsequently, obstruction of the left gastric vein and short gastric veins results in the formation of gastroesophageal varices (GOV). Approximately 50% of cirrhotic patients present with GOV, and the severity of GOV is closely correlated with the severity of cirrhosis. Endoscopy serves as the gold standard for the diagnosis of GOV [16]. The presence and grades of GOV can be determined *via* endoscopic examination, thus guiding therapeutic intervention in clinical practice. For cirrhotic patients without GOV, a repeat gastroscopic examination every 2–3 years is recommended, whereas for those suffering from GOV, a repeat endoscopic examination every 1–2 years is recommended.

2.2 Primary prophylaxis of esophageal variceal bleeding (EVB)

The objective of primary prophylaxis for EVB is to eliminate the underlying causes, lessen the degree of varices, prevent bleeding, and reduce the occurrence of other complications. Different approaches are adopted based on the severity of esophageal varices. Currently, nonselective beta-blockers (NSBBs) and endoscopic variceal ligation (EVL) are preferred methods for primary prophylaxis of esophageal varices, with carvedilol showing significant efficacy among NSBBs [17]. For cirrhotic patients without esophageal varices or with small varices, NSBBs are not recommended for prevention, except for those at higher bleeding risk from small varices. In patients with moderate to large varices, both NSBBs and endoscopic treatments are recommended. For those who cannot tolerate NSBBs, EVL is the preferred option to prevent the first episode bleeding. A meta-analysis of 19 randomized controlled trials indicated no significant difference between the EVL and NSBB groups in terms of bleeding and mortality [18]. EVL should be performed every 2–4 weeks until varices eradication, with follow-up every 3–6 months within the first year. Research on primary prevention for GOV is limited. Currently, primary prophylaxis for GOV1 is similar to that for esophageal varices (EV), while for GOV2 and isolated gastric varices (IGV) 1, the AASLD and the European Association for the Study of the Liver (EASL) recommend NSBB. Endoscopic variceal obturation (EVO), echoendoscopy-guided coil insertion, and balloon-occluded retrograde transvenous obliteration (BRTO) are feasible options. The combination of EVL and NSBB is not recommended.

2.3 Treatment of acute esophageal variceal bleeding (AEVB)

Acute esophageal variceal bleeding (AEVB) represents a prevalent and life-threatening complication among patients with liver cirrhosis, accounting for approximately one-third of mortality in this population. Consequently, managing AEVB is of critical importance. The main treatments include early management, pharmacotherapy, endoscopy, and rescue therapy. Early management principles primarily involve maintaining airway patency, fluid resuscitation, and controlling infection. There is ongoing debate regarding the necessity of Sengstaken-Blakemore tube prior to endoscopic examination or treatment in patients with AEVB. Pharmacotherapy is the preferred treatment for AEVB. Prompt initiation of treatment aimed at reducing portal venous pressure and controlling infection is crucial. Commonly used medications to decrease portal venous pressure include terlipressin, somatostatin, and octreotide. Studies indicate that 20% of cirrhosis patients with active bleeding will develop bacterial infection within 48 hours, underscoring the critical importance of infection prevention [19]. Current guidelines recommend short-term antibiotic prophylaxis (5–7 days), with intravenous ceftriaxone at a dosage of 1–2 g/day being the preferred agent [15, 17, 20, 21].Gastroscopy is the primary treatment for diagnosing and managing AEVB. According to AASLD and EASL guidelines, patients with AEVB should undergo endoscopic examination within 12 hours, whereas APASL advises the timing of endoscopic examination should be within 6 hours. Endoscopic treatment options include endoscopic variceal ligation (EVL), endoscopic injection sclerotherapy (EIS), and endoscopic injection of tissue adhesives. EVL is recommended as the first-line treatment for patients with EV and type 1 gastroesophageal varices (GOV1). Endoscopic injection of tissue adhesives is primarily utilized for patients with bleeding from IGV and GOV2. Studies have shown that the efficacy of EVL and tissue adhesive injection in treating active bleeding is comparable, but the rebleeding rate in patients treated with tissue adhesive injection is significantly lower than that in patients treated with EVL [19]. Transjugular intrahepatic portosystemic shunt (TIPS) is the preferred treatment for patients who remain bleeding after drug or endoscopic therapy. Balloon-occluded retrograde transvenous obliteration (BRTO), which obstructs abnormal shunts *via* a balloon catheter, targets GOV2, IGV1, and varices at rare sites and is suitable for patients with or at high risk of hepatic encephalopathy.

2.4 Secondary prevention of EVB

The objective of secondary prevention is to avert the recurrence of bleeding from esophagogastric varices. Typically, secondary prevention measures are initiated for patients with a history of EVB or 5 days after treatment for AEVB. A Hepatic Venous Pressure Gradient (HVPG) >20 mmHg serves as an early predictor of rebleeding.

For patients with EV bleeding, the combination of NSBBs and EVL is recommended for secondary prevention. The dosage for NSBBs remains the same as for primary prevention, while EVL is recommended every 1–4 weeks until varices are obliterated. For GOV1 bleeding, due to limited research, recommendations align with those for EV. The American Association for the Study of Liver Diseases (AASLD) suggests NSBBs and EVL (or Endoscopic Variceal Obliteration, EVO) as secondary preventive measures, while the Korean Association for the Study of the Liver (KASL) advocates repeated use of EVO or EVL. For GOV2 and IGV1 bleeding, the AASLD recommends TIPS or BRTO as secondary prevention, whereas KASL suggests EVO or BRTO. Given the absence of unified protocols, secondary prevention should be personalized based on the patient's specific circumstances and local healthcare resources.

3. Management of ascites

For cirrhotic patients suffer ascites, abstinence from alcohol and treatment of the underlying cause are strongly recommended. Etiological treatment can alleviate liver fibrosis, reduce portal vein pressure, and reverse the progression of liver fibrosis and cirrhosis. For patients unable to undergo etiological treatment, interventions such as antifibrotic therapy, prevention of intestinal bacterial translocation, protection of endothelial cell function, and correction of coagulation abnormalities can also improve the progression of complications. Cirrhotic patients with ascites should focus on nutritional balance to prevent malnutrition. Early detection, diagnosis, and treatment of nutritional deficiencies are crucial. Guidelines recommend small, frequent meals, bedtime snacks, and supplementation with branched-chain amino acids. Moderate salt restriction is beneficial for the alleviation of ascites. The Asia-Pacific Association and the British Society of Gastroenterology along with the British Association for the Study [22, 23] of the Liver suggest a salt intake of 5–6.5 g/L for patients with ascites, while in China, the recommended intake is 4–6 g/L. However, it is essential to be cautious of the risk of hyponatremia (<110 mmol/L) with restricted salt diets.

Albumin plays a vital physiological role in management of ascites. Guidelines recommend supplementing 6–8 g of albumin per 1000 ml of ascites removed, which could significantly increase patients' survival rates [24]. Diuretics are classified into aldosterone antagonists (spironolactone), loop diuretics (furosemide), and vasopressin V2 receptor antagonists (tolvaptan) according to different mechanisms. Diuretics and its dosage selection is based on the grades of ascites. For patients with grade 1 ascites, spironolactone may be prescribed alone initially, with the option to increase the dose or combine with furosemide if ineffective. For patients with grade 2–3 ascites, it is advised to administrate with a combination of spironolactone and furosemide, monitoring urine output and ascites volume. Large volume paracentesis (LVP) is an effective treatment strategy for grade 3 ascites, refractory ascites, and recurrent ascites. It is essential to administer albumin to counterbalance fluid removal and maintain colloid osmotic pressure during LVP. Transjugular intrahepatic portosystemic shunt (TIPS) is one of the primary treatment strategies for refractory or recurrent ascites and can also serve as a bridging therapy to liver transplantation or as the preferred treatment for patients who are not suitable for transplantation. For cirrhotic patients who is classified with Child-Pugh C or complicating with liver failure, liver transplantation should be considered as a priority treatment. And efforts should be made to minimize the risk of infections for pretransplantation.

4. Spontaneous bacterial peritonitis (SBP)

SBP is a common complication in patients with end-stage liver cirrhosis. Immediate empirical antibiotic therapy is essential upon SBP suspicion, adjusting based on the results of bacterial culture of ascites. Empirical antibiotic treatment depends on whether SBP is community-acquired or hospital-acquired. For community-acquired SBP, treatment primarily targets Gram-negative bacilli, with third-generation cephalosporins (e.g., cefotaxime) as the first choice. Carbapenems are preferred for broad-spectrum coverage in areas with high antimicrobial resistance rates. Piperacillin/tazobactam is chosen in regions with lower resistance rates, while carbapenems are favored in high-resistance areas. The duration of antibiotic administration should be at least 5–7 days. Consensus suggests administering albumin to patients with SBP can reduce drug clearance, significantly enhance anti-infection effects, and improve patients' survival. Albumin dosage should be administered of 1.5 g/kg within 6 hours on the first day, followed by 1 g/kg on the third day [25]. For SBP prevention, cirrhotic patients with variceal bleeding should receive prophylactic treatment. Patients with low ascitic fluid protein (<1.5 g/L) are at higher risk for SBP. Those with severe liver disease (Child-Pugh score $\geq$ 9 with serum bilirubin $\geq$3 mg/dL) or renal impairment (serum creatinine $\geq$1.2 mg/dL, blood urea nitrogen $\geq$25 mg/dL, or serum sodium $\leq$130 mq/L) should receive antibiotic prophylaxis for primary SBP prevention. Long-term prophylactic treatment with oral norfloxacin, ciprofloxacin, or trimethoprim-sulfamethoxazole after correction of SBP is recommended [26].

5. Hepatic encephalopathy (HE)

Hepatic encephalopathy (HE) is a neuropsychiatric syndrome of varying severity, resulting from severe liver dysfunction or various abnormalities in the portal-systemic circulation. It is characterized by metabolic disruptions and neurological and psychiatric abnormalities of differing degrees. HE represents a common complication and cause of mortality in severe liver diseases [27]. The West-Haven classification is the most commonly utilized clinical classification system for HE, categorizing HE into grades 0, 1, 2, 3, and 4. According to the SONIC grading criteria, grades 0 and 1 HE are classified as covert hepatic encephalopathy (CHE), while grades 2, 3, and 4 HE are defined as overt hepatic encephalopathy (OHE). OHE is further subdivided into episodic, recurrent, and persistent based on the course of HE. Recurrent HE refers to episodes occurring within a 6-month interval, whereas persistent HE denotes sustained behavioral alterations with no recovery between two episodes, interspersed with recurrences of overt HE. CHE is considered as a risk factor for OHE; thus, treating CHE is a preventative measure for OHE [28]. Research [29] indicates that 30–45% of patients with cirrhosis experience OHE, with an annual incidence rate of 20%. Following TIPS placement, the occurrence rate can escalate to as high as 50%. Blood ammonia levels could be used for the diagnosis of HE, although levels can be high, low, or even asymptomatic [30]. Structural MRI can also be utilized to differentiate HE from other diseases [31]. Treatment principles include removing precipitating factors, nutritional support therapy, and individualized treatment. Lactulose is considered the first-line therapy for all patients with HE, reducing the incidence of OHE and improving cognitive function. Rifaximin, a poorly absorbed antibiotic, is recommended when lactulose fails to prevent recurrent HE episodes. Rifaximin has been proven to reduce the risk of HE recurrence and rehospitalization and improve quality of life. However, the debate between monotherapy and combination therapy for preventing HE recurrence remains contentious and requires further investigation. The use of proton pump inhibitors (PPIs) should be carefully reassessed in patients with cirrhosis due to their potential to increase the incidence of HE [32].

6. Hepatorenal syndrome (HRS)

HRS is a functional renal failure that occurs in patients with advanced liver disease. It is characterized by renal functional impairment, significant alterations in hemodynamics, and marked abnormalities in endogenous vasoactive substances. The exact mechanism of HRS remains unclear, but it is often attributed to severe liver dysfunction leading to hemodynamic changes, severe renal hypoperfusion, decreased renal blood flow, and subsequent renal functional failure. The treatment of HRS involves general measures, pharmacotherapy, and others. General treatment measures include early administration of a high-calorie easily digestible diet, monitoring of blood pressure, urine output, and liver and kidney function. Maintaining fluid balance to prevent fluid overload and dilutional hyponatremia is crucial. Aggressive infection control is also recommended. Pharmacotherapy includes albumin and vasoconstrictor drugs such as norepinephrine, terlipressin, and midodrine combined with octreotide. Guidelines recommend albumin replacement therapy for hepatorenal syndrome-acute kidney injury (HRS-AKI) patients with serum creatinine levels >1.5 mg/dL (132.6 μmol/L). Vasoconstrictor therapy, particularly terlipressin, is recommended for all HRS-AKI patients in combination with intravenous albumin infusion. Terlipressin is administered initially at 2 mg/d continuous infusion, up to a maximum of 12 mg/d, until AKI reversal. In China, the protocol involves terlipressin (1 mg every 4–6 hours) combined with albumin (20–40 g/d) for 3 days, with adjustments based on serum creatinine levels. If terlipressin is ineffective, somatostatin analogs or norepinephrine combined with albumin can be tried as alternative treatments. Liver transplantation is the preferred treatment for HRS-AKI patients, while there is limited evidence to support the use of TIPS and blood purification therapy for HRS. These treatments may be considered in select cases but are not universally recommended.

In conclusion, the timely identification and treatment of cirrhosis and its complications are paramount. Managing cirrhosis is a multidisciplinary endeavor that necessitates the creation of personalized treatment strategies tailored to each patient's unique situation. As our understanding of the disease mechanisms deepens and treatment modalities continue to advance, there is optimism for further enhancements in patient outcomes. By implementing comprehensive management approaches and staying abreast of emerging therapeutic innovations, we can strive to optimize the care and prognosis of individuals affected by cirrhosis.

Author details

Zhenyu Wu*, Lei Chen*, Jing Chen and Chuanfang Chen
Department of Gastroenterology, The First Affiliated Hospital (Southwest Hospital) to Third Military Medical University (Army Medical University), Chongqing, China

*Address all correspondence to: wuzy9204@163.com and chenlei_1977603@126.com

References

[1] European Association for the Study of the Liver. EASL clinical practice guidelines on the management of hepatic encephalopathy. Journal of Hepatology. 2022;**77**(3):807-824

[2] Roberto DF, Jaime B, Guadalupe G-T, et al. Baveno VII—Renewing consensus in portal hypertension. Journal of Hepatology. 2022;**76**(4):959-974

[3] Yoshiji H, Nagoshi S, Akahane T, et al. Evidence-based clinical practice guidelines for liver cirrhosis 2020. Journal of Gastroenterology. 2021;**56**(7):593-619

[4] Ginès P, Krag A, Abraldes JG, et al. Liver cirrhosis. Lancet. 2021;**398**(10308):1359-1376

[5] Jalan R, D'Amico G, Trebicka J, et al. New clinical and pathophysiological perspectives defining the trajectory of cirrhosis. Journal of Hepatology. 2021;**75**(Suppl 1):S14-s26

[6] Choi C, Choi DH, Spears GM, et al. Relationship between etiology of cirrhosis and survival among patients hospitalized in intensive care units. Mayo Clinic Proceedings. 2022;**97**(2):274-284

[7] Kim TH, Um SH, Lee YS, et al. Determinants of re-compensation in patients with hepatitis B virus-related decompensated cirrhosis starting antiviral therapy. Alimentary Pharmacology & Therapeutics. 2022;**55**(1):83-96

[8] Kisseleva T, Brenner D. Molecular and cellular mechanisms of liver fibrosis and its regression. Nature Reviews. Gastroenterology & Hepatology. 2021;**18**(3):151-166

[9] Gentile I, Scotto R, Coppola C, et al. Treatment with direct-acting antivirals improves the clinical outcome in patients with HCV-related decompensated cirrhosis: Results from an Italian real-life cohort (liver network activity-LINA cohort). Hepatology International. 2019;**13**(1):66-74

[10] Cai X, Liu X, Xie W, et al. Hydronidone for the treatment of liver fibrosis related to chronic hepatitis B: A phase 2 randomized controlled trial. Clinical Gastroenterology and Hepatology. 2023;**21**(7):1893-1901.e1897

[11] Zeng X, Tang XJ, Sheng X, et al. Does low-dose rifaximin ameliorate endotoxemia in patients with liver cirrhosis: A prospective study. Journal of Digestive Diseases. 2015;**16**(11):665-674

[12] Pose E, Napoleone L, Amin A, et al. Safety of two different doses of simvastatin plus rifaximin in decompensated cirrhosis (LIVERHOPE-SAFETY): A randomised, double-blind, placebo-controlled, phase 2 trial. The Lancet Gastroenterology & Hepatology. 2020;**5**(1):31-41

[13] Muñoz AE, Pollarsky FD, Marino M, et al. Addition of statins to the standard treatment in patients with cirrhosis: Safety and efficacy. World Journal of Gastroenterology. 2021;**27**(28):4639-4652

[14] European Association for the Study of the Liver. Electronic address:easloffice@easloffice.eu. EASL clinical practice guidelines on nutrition in chronic liver disease. Journal of Hepatology. 2019;**70**(1):172-193

[15] European Association for the Study of the Liver. Electronic address:easloffice@easloffice.eu.

EASL clinical practice guidelines for the management of patients with decompensated cirrhosis. Journal of Hepatology. 2018;**69**(2):406-460

[16] Hwang JH, Shergill AK, Acosta RD, et al. The role of endoscopy in the management of variceal hemorrhage. Gastrointestinal Endoscopy. 2014;**80**(2):221-227

[17] Korean Association for the Study of the Liver (KASL). KASL clinical practice guidelines for liver cirrhosis: Varices, hepatic encephalopathy, and related complications. Clinical and Molecular Hepatology. 2020;**26**(2):83-127

[18] Funakoshi N, Duny Y, Valats JC, et al. Meta-analysis: Beta-blockers versus banding ligation for primary prophylaxis of esophageal variceal bleeding. Annals of Hepatology. 2012;**11**(3):369-383

[19] Tapper EB, Parikh ND. Diagnosis and Management of Cirrhosis and its Complications: A review. Journal of the American Medical Association. 2023;**329**(18):1589-1602

[20] Garcia-Tsao G, Abraldes JG, Berzigotti A, et al. Portal hypertensive bleeding in cirrhosis: Risk stratification, diagnosis, and management: 2016 practice guidance by the American association for the study of liver diseases. Hepatology. 2017;**65**(1):310-335

[21] Sarin SK, Kumar A, Angus PW, et al. Diagnosis and management of acute variceal bleeding: Asian Pacific Association for Study of the liver recommendations. Hepatology International. 2011;**5**(2):607-624

[22] Singh V, De A, Mehtani R, et al. Asia-Pacific association for study of liver guidelines on management of ascites in liver disease. Hepatology International. 2023;**17**(4):792-826

[23] Aithal GP, Palaniyappan N, China L, et al. Guidelines on the management of ascites in cirrhosis. Gut. 2021;**70**(1):9-29

[24] Biggins SW, Angeli P, Garcia-Tsao G, et al. Diagnosis, evaluation, and Management of Ascites, spontaneous bacterial peritonitis and Hepatorenal syndrome: 2021 practice guidance by the American Association for the Study of Liver Diseases. Hepatology. 2021;**74**(2):1014-1048

[25] Kim SW, Yoon JS, Park J, et al. Empirical treatment with Carbapenem vs third-generation cephalosporin for treatment of spontaneous bacterial peritonitis. Clinical Gastroenterology and Hepatology. 2021;**19**(5):976-986.e975

[26] Praharaj DL, Premkumar M, Roy A, et al. Norfloxacin for spontaneous bacterial peritonitis prophylaxis: A randomized controlled trial. Journal of Clinical and Experimental Hepatology. 2022;**12**(2):336-342

[27] Hepatic encephalopathy in chronic liver disease. 2014 practice guideline by the European Association for the Study of the liver and the American Association for the Study of Liver Diseases. Journal of Hepatology. 2014;**61**(3):642-659

[28] Zacharias HD, Kamel F, Tan J, et al. Rifaximin for prevention and treatment of hepatic encephalopathy in people with cirrhosis. Cochrane Database of Systematic Reviews. 2023;**7**(7):Cd011585

[29] Bajaj JS. Review article: The modern management of hepatic encephalopathy. Alimentary Pharmacology & Therapeutics. 2010;**31**(5):537-547

[30] Rahimi RS, Safadi R, Thabut D, et al. Efficacy and Safety of ornithine Phenylacetate for treating overt hepatic encephalopathy in a randomized

trial. Clinical Gastroenterology and Hepatology. 2021;**19**(12):2626-2635.e2627

[31] Rovira A, Alonso J, Córdoba J. MR imaging findings in hepatic encephalopathy. AJNR. American Journal of Neuroradiology. 2008;**29**(9):1612-1621

[32] Sharma BC, Sharma P, Lunia MK, et al. A randomized, double-blind, controlled trial comparing rifaximin plus lactulose with lactulose alone in treatment of overt hepatic encephalopathy. The American Journal of Gastroenterology. 2013;**108**(9):1458-1463